T0146772

Love Yoga

*Two people with a desire for
yoga and each other*

LISA PERRIS

BALBOA.
PRESS
A DIVISION OF HAY HOUSE

Balboa Press books may be ordered through booksellers or by contacting:

Balboa Press
A Division of Hay House
1663 Liberty Drive
Bloomington, IN 47403
www.balboapress.com
1 (877) 407-4847

Because of the dynamic nature of the Internet, any web addresses or links contained in this book may have changed since publication and may no longer be valid. The views expressed in this work are solely those of the author and do not necessarily reflect the views of the publisher, and the publisher hereby disclaims any responsibility for them.

The author of this book does not dispense medical advice or prescribe the use of any technique as a form of treatment for physical, emotional, or medical problems without the advice of a physician, either directly or indirectly. The intent of the author is only to offer information of a general nature to help you in your quest for emotional and spiritual well-being. In the event you use any of the information in this book for yourself, which is your constitutional right, the author and the publisher assume no responsibility for your actions.

Any people depicted in stock imagery provided by Thinkstock are models, and such images are being used for illustrative purposes only. Certain stock imagery © Thinkstock.

Print information available on the last page.

ISBN: 978-1-5043-2768-8 (sc)
ISBN: 978-1-5043-2770-1 (hc)
ISBN: 978-1-5043-2769-5 (e)

Library of Congress Control Number: 2015902117

Balboa Press rev. date: 04/15/2015

The practical guide to yoga postures combined with love making. If you believe you are having a spiritual journey, then trust in the gift of yoga to help you on your path. If you believe in love, then treasure the gift of every moment together, because life is short and kinship is precious.

Contents

Part One - The Practical Yoga Handbook

What Is Yoga? 3
Contraindications of Yoga and Safe Sex 5
Health Benefits of Yoga 7

The Breath 9
Breathing Techniques (Pranayama) 11
Abdominal Breathing 14
Victorious Breath (Ujjayi) 15
Alternate Nostril Breathing (Anuloma Viloma) 16

Opening Poses 19
Cobbler Pose (Baddha Konasana) 20
Pigeon Pose (Kapotasana) 24

Sequence Work and Transition Poses 27
Sun Salutation (Surya Namaskar) 28
Downward Facing Dog Pose (Adho Mukha Svanasana) 32
Plank Pose (Kumbhakasana) 36

Standing Poses 39
Crescent Moon Pose (Anjaneyasana) 40
Wide Leg Standing Forward Bend Pose (Prasarita Padottanasana) 44
Triangle Pose (Trikonasana) 48
Warrior I Pose (Virabhadrasana I) 52

Twisting Pose 55
Half Spinal Twist Pose (Ardha Matsyendrasana) 56

Balance Poses 59
Tree Pose (Vrksasana) 60
Extended Hand to Big Toe Pose (Utthita Hasta Padangusthasana) 64
Lord Shiva's Pose or Dancer Pose (Natarajasana) 68

Crow Pose (Khakasana)...72
Boat Pose (Navasana)...76

Inversion Poses...79
Shoulder Stand Pose (Sarvangasana).................................80
Plough Pose (Halasana)...84

Inversion Counter Pose...87
Fish Pose (Matsyasana)...88

Backward Bend Poses 91
Bridge Pose (Setu Bandhasana Sarvangasana).........................92
Wheel Pose (Chakrasana) 96
Cobra Pose (Bhujangasana) 100
Camel Pose (Ustrasana) 104

Forward Bend Pose 107
Legs Spread Back Stretch Pose (Pada Prasar Paschimottanasana) .. 108

Relaxation Poses 111
Extended Swan Pose (Utthita Hamsasana).............................112
Easy Pose (Sukhasana) 114
Corpse Pose (Savasana) 116

Part Two - Setting the Mood

Make the Connection 123
Chakras..125
Love to Meditate 133

Sensory Pleasure...135
Visual...137
Talk (and Listen) 139
Touch..142
Smell 145
Taste..146

Part Three - Creating the Union of Love

The Entwined Collection – Two People with a Desire for
Yoga and Each Other..151

Foreplay 153
#1 Crow and Corpse Pose 155
#2 Boat and Cobra Pose 156
#3 Tree and Mountain Pose 157
#4 Mountain and Shoulder Stand Pose 158
#5 Crescent Moon and Easy Pose..................................... 159
#6 Extended Hand to Big Toe and Easy Pose 160
#7 Camel and Cobra Pose 161

Sexual Connection.. 163
#8 Pigeon and Easy Pose 165
#9 Dancer and Mountain Pose.. 166
#10 Shoulder Stand and Warrior I Pose............................. 167
#11 The Cobbler Combination... 168
#12 Bridge Pose 169
#13 Triangle Pose (Both Parties)...................................... 170
#14 Wheel and Mountain Pose 171
#15 Warrior Creation 172
#16 Downward Facing Dog (Extended Leg) and Warrior I Pose......... 173
#17 Corpse and Plank Pose..174
#18 Cobbler and Plank Pose... 175
#19 Forward Bend and Mountain Pose 176
#20 Legs Spread Back Stretch Pose (Both Parties) 177
#21 Boat and Cobra Pose... 178
#22 Corpse and Legs Spread Back Stretch Pose (Reversed)............ 179
#23 Mountain and Extended Hand to Big Toe Pose 180

1

The Practical Yoga Handbook

What Is Yoga?

One translation for yoga is *union,* which is an apt meaning for this book. We create a union by connecting our mind, body, breath and spirit within oneself, and a union with other human beings, particularly our soul mates and lovers.

Yoga is an ancient art form devised to provide an individual person with a healthy spirit, mind, and body. Although the journey to enlightenment is a long one – and probably one that we will never reach in our lifetime – it is never too late to appreciate the health benefits gifted to us through yoga.

Through a series of physical poses which help to focus the mind, and by focusing on the breath whilst participating in posture work, the spirit reaches out for enlightenment. This takes many years of practice, and most of us never reach that goal, but striving towards the goal will make your life more fulfilled and healthy.

The series of postures and techniques have been around for thousands of years and derives from India. It has been changed and modified, and the array of poses has increased as different parties added their own interpretations and philosophies. Today yoga is practised throughout the world and is accepted as a very positive form of exercise for general well-being.

By combining yoga and love making, this sense of fulfilment is heightened and shared with another. This combination has long been around, if you take for example the Karma Sutra. This book is a simplified version, showing how amazing postures can be combined together and used to create one harmonious action.

A yoga session is practised by blending breathing and relaxation techniques along with pose combinations, which can include a composed selection of forward bends, back bends, an inversion along with a counter pose, balance, and twist postures. Often included is a sequence or series arrangement, such as the sun salutation.

Yoga is about being in the present moment. Connect to the here and now. Stop thinking about the past; you cannot change anything because it has gone, and the future is yet to arrive, so enjoy now.

Whilst yoga has varied meanings in different writings, the main focus should be what it actually means to you. Every time I practise, I feel life force surging energetically through my body, the chatter in my brain is quieter, and I am more open and aware of others. The positive elements in my life seem enhanced, my focus is greater, my body moves more fluidly, I breathe more deeply as my chest is open, and my spirit feels nourished. These are merely my feelings, but do take time to think about your experience and what yoga means to you.

Contraindications of Yoga and Safe Sex

Yoga is something that can be experienced on your own or as part of a class, or if you choose to do so, you could partake as a couple with the possibility that it may bring you closer together. If you have not undertaken yoga previously, then please consider attending a class before participating in a home practice; this will ensure correct posture alignment under the watchful eye of a qualified instructor.

Do not attempt to do yoga if you have had a recent operation or if you are pregnant, unless you are an experienced practitioner and have taken advice as to the postures you can and cannot do. This book has not been designed for women who are pregnant even though it may refer to pregnancy in certain text.

If you have medical conditions such as high or low blood pressure, heart problems, a hernia, glaucoma, liver problems, diabetes, lung disorders, breathing issues, or abdominal pain; or if you suffer from epilepsy, ulcers, vertigo; or if you have acute back conditions, then seek medical advice before attempting any of the techniques outlined within this book. If you are suffering or recovering from a cold, or if you have sinus issues, the flu, or a chest infection, do not undertake any exercise. Ensure that you are fully recovered before participating in any form of training.

If you are medicated for any conditions outlined above and have them fully under control, then it may be perfectly acceptable to undertake a yoga practice. However, in all cases it is imperative to seek medical advice and receive full clearance to participate. If you have an illness or condition that may not be listed above, it is always important to consult your GP and get consent before you exercise.

Injury can occur if the postures are carried out incorrectly. Use an aid if needed; for example, if you find it difficult to balance, then use a chair or wall to hold on to because this will help with centering yourself as you carry out the pose.

Do not exercise if you have had a heavy meal, consumed alcohol, or are intoxicated with drugs, even if you feel that you are able to do so. If you feel unwell at any point, stop immediately and seek medical advice. Always ensure that you are fully hydrated, and do not hold a posture if it feels uncomfortable or if you are straining to do so. Work within the parameters of your own health and well-being, and at all times listen to your body because it is the best indicator of your physical condition.

Always seek medical advice. It is your own responsibility to ensure that you are safe and well enough to participate in anything outlined within this book. Read each element carefully before attempting anything.

Safe Sex

It is imperative to protect yourself under all circumstances against sexually transmitted diseases. Use suitable contraception to avoid pregnancy, assuming a potential new addition to the family is not desired at this point.

Health Benefits of Yoga

By undertaking the yoga postures correctly during your practice, you will gain tremendous benefit. The poses do not need to look perfect like something out of a book. Carrying out the postures effectively means that they should suit your bodies' capabilities and limitations. Yoga is not a competition with others or yourself; it is something to be experienced in the moment and enjoyed for all its health benefits. Appreciate your capabilities in the present moment. Do not force the body because that will create adverse affects.

Through practice you may become more flexible and have a calmer, clearer mind. You will experience a sense of relaxation whilst achieving mental clarity and greater focus. The muscles in your body will become toned, and your cells will be oxygenated. Inside the body the benefits are endless too. More oxygen will flow around the body, and the endocrine, digestive, and circulatory systems will function more effectively as toxins are expelled from the body. Deep, rhythmic breathing is encouraged.

Physical

It tones the internal organs and external muscles of the body, creating better alignment, enhancing flexibility, balancing the equilibrium, and combating physical issues such as obesity.

Mental

Yoga can be very calming for the mind, soothing brain chatter (this is the feeling you get when your mind is in overdrive, and you are struggling to quiet it down). The thought process becomes clearer, concentration is improved, and focus is resumed.

Spiritual

Not everyone believes in the connection to our spiritual selves, and I appreciate that *Love Yoga* will be used by a variety of people. Some people will want to experience the spiritual side of yoga and meditation, but others won't. This could be a beginning source of information to start that journey before moving onto further literature to expand your knowledge on spiritual development. A spiritual path is a personal choice. Others will use yoga to simply get physically fit, and by using *Love Yoga* they will gain the added benefit of combining yoga with a physical and mental connection to their partners on a sexual level. Whatever way you want to experience this book, it is your choice.

Fundamentally, all human beings are the same and are connected on a soul level. Souls do not recognise sexual preference, gender, race, creed, or disability – only love and the good in one another. Unfortunately, the human thought process sometimes clouds this and brings about negativity towards others. All living creatures have a soul, and that makes us individuals. When we cease to exist on earth, some people believe that our soul-life journey continues on an alternative plane (another dimension). It goes on a progressive journey in development, moving further along the path to enlightenment. The contrasting view to this is that when the physical body dies, then so does the soul; our entire being diminishes, and we are no more.

You do not have to be religious to be spiritual – not that I frown upon any type or religion or personal belief system. We are given the freedom of choice and the ability of acceptance, but throughout our lives we can sometimes be influenced by others. Be true to who you are and trust in your own spiritual journey; let this book enhance the enjoyment along the way by connecting you with yourself on a deeper level and your chosen life partner through intimacy and love.

All of these ingredients combined will aid a healthier, more balanced, enjoyable life. You will find new love for yourself and your partner, bringing you closer together on your life path.

The Breath

Breathing Techniques (Pranayama)

Why is the breath key to good yoga practice?

> As long as there is breath in the body, there is life. When breath departs so too does life. Therefore regulate the breath.
>
> – Hatha Yoga Pradipika

Pranayama, or breathing exercises, are the key to yoga. It is through the practice of Pranayama that the mind becomes still and finds peace. Even though breathing is an automatic function, it is likely that it is being carried out incorrectly, and the lungs are not being used to their full capacity, which affects your optimum health. Through the practise of breathing exercises, we learn to take control of the breath, making our bodies function more efficiently and giving us a healthier life.

Prana translates to 'life force', and yama is 'discipline' or 'control'. Ayama means 'expansion', 'non-restraint', or 'extension'. These make up the word Pranayama, meaning 'breathing techniques'. The breath is the transportation system for carrying prana. Prana is our life force, known as Qui or Chi.

Without breath we would cease to exist. In yoga, breathing is the link between the mind and body. It brings them both together by assisting a practitioner with postures; as we focus on the breath, we forget how difficult the pose may be to hold, and therefore it acts as a welcome distraction and aids our practice. It helps to connect a person into the moment and provides energy to hold strong, physical poses whilst offering calmness to the mind.

To avoid losing prana and to help keep it concentrated within a specific area of the physical body, we can apply something known as bandhas, which means 'to be binding' (bondage). To lock a bandha, it is necessary, whilst in a posture, to contract particular muscles depending on which lock we require. This creates a psycho-muscular energy lock, redirecting the flow of prana.

When you are experiencing times of stress or are in a demanding, hectic situation, yoga advises you to breathe. You do this because it brings clarity to a busy, anxious mind and offers you peace and a moment to think clearly and reflect.

Pranayama practice has a very important purpose because it ensures that the respiratory system is working to its full potential. The breath provides the body with essential oxygenation, helping with the regeneration of cells; this occurs in the flow of respiration. When the respiratory system is working to its full capacity, other systems of the body benefit as well. The circulatory system improves, which in turn aids the digestive system, assisting the body in the elimination of destructive toxins and preventing accumulation of negative blockages. Our respiratory system is essential to purifying our bodies and minds. The main ingredient of yoga which enables this to occur is the practice of Pranayama.

The practise of Pranayama assists in cleansing the nadis, which are the energy lines of the subtle body. There are 72,000 nadis within the subtle body, and the majority of these start around the navel and heart centre. The practise of breathing techniques ensures the optimum health of the nadis, which in turn changes the attitude of sadhaka (our spiritual path for self-realisation, true reality, and cosmic consciousness).

This occurs because Pranayama breathing starts at the base of the diaphragm, which is situated on each side of the body near to the pelvic girdle. When we breathe deeply using this part of the diaphragm, the thoracic diaphragm and the respiratory muscles of the neck are relaxed, which subsequently rest the facial muscles. When the face muscles are relaxed, they slacken their grip on the vital organs of perception – the eyes, tongue, nose, and ears – which eases tension in the brain, allowing the sadhaka to attain awareness and to be composed and serene.

There four stages of Pranayama are (1) commencement (arambha), (2) intent endeavour (ghata), (3) intimate knowledge (parichaya), and (4) consummation (nispatti).

Continued and regular practice of Pranayama helps us to break down the various barriers of each level and move through the stages from awakening, to hopefully reaching the stage of ecstasy (enlightenment).

Abdominal Breathing

Prana (Chi), our life force, needs to move freely around the body in order to provide us with energy. The prana moves in and out of the subtle body just as we inhale and exhale air in the physical body.

Description

This type of breathing brings focus to the movement of the breath; it is the first stage of breath control. It is important to a person's yoga practice to get the breathing correct at the early stages, because many of us breathe incorrectly. Due to tension and the stresses of life, most of us do not know how to relax the stomach and the diaphragm; we only use the chest to breathe. This is called shallow breathing, and it is a bad habit that needs to be transformed.

The Practice

Lie on the floor or yoga mat in corpse pose (savasana) with the eyes closed. Gently rest the hands on the abdomen, allowing the tips of the fingers to touch. Breathe in and out through the nostrils.

As you inhale and the body fills with air, inflate the abdomen, pushing the hands away. On the exhalation, the stomach flattens and the air is expelled from the body.

It takes time to get this practise right, especially if you have been habitually breathing incorrectly for a considerable length of time.

It is natural during the practice for the mind to have a tendency to wander to other subjects. Whilst this is normal, it is imperative to regularly bring the mind back to focus on the breath. Observe as it gently enters and exits the body.

Victorious Breath (Ujjayi)

Ujjayi breathing is the second stage of breath control, following the accomplishment of abdominal breathing. The Sanskrit of 'uj' means expand, and 'jayai' means victory.

Description

The Ujjayi breath is a cleansing and soothing breath known as a Kriya. It removes mucus from the throat, clearing the throat chakra (vishudda), which assists with communication, speech, and emotional liberation. It is only suitable for beginner students to practise this style of breathing on an out breath, which encourages a full exhalation before inhaling again normally. More advanced students can use the Ujjayi breath for both the inhalation and exhalation. It encourages a complete breath.

The Practice

This practice can be carried out either near the start or end of a session, for five to ten minutes. It can also be carried out throughout the practice if you are an accomplished yoga student. Whilst lying on the floor with the eyes closed and continuing to observe the breath as it enters and exits the nostrils, bring attention to the throat. Ujjayi breathing creates an audiable sound by slightly constricting the back of the throat, and by partly closing the epiglottis and restricting the air flow whilst still breathing in and out through the nose. This noise gives the mind something to focus on, and it ensures that you as the practitioner stay in the moment. It can be carried out in a seated position as well as during asana practise. Ensure that the inhalation and exhalation are elongated.

Alternate Nostril Breathing (Anuloma Viloma)

Description

Alternate nostril breathing is practised to create balance in the mind and body with a calming affect. The right nostril is connected with pingala, and the left nostril is connected with ida: these are activated and harmonised during this practise. This is a breathing technique that controls the inhalation and exhalation.

Before practising this technique, it is essential that you are first fully acquainted with the natural abdominal breathing process. Breathing exercises are usually performed at the beginning of a practice because they assist in calming the mind, bringing energy into the body, and connecting the body and mind together in preparation for a session.

The Practice

Sit on your yoga mat in a comfortable, cross-legged position. If this is not comfortable, then it is acceptable to sit on your knees or sit with the legs stretched out in front of you, depending on which is the most suitable for your needs. Ensure that your back is straight and your chin is parallel to the ground. Always use the right hand to control the nasal passages, even if you are left handed. In yoga the right side is generally activated first. It is the side which is the masculine, solar, active and positive elements whilst the opposing left side is feminine, lunar, inactive and negative side.

Place the left hand in Chin Mudra (A) and the right hand in Vishnu Mudra (B).

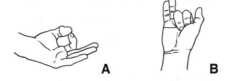

Rest the left hand facing upwards on the left knee. The right hand is the active hand. When taking part in the practice, the right elbow is not to be held directly in front of the chest because this restricts the breath.

The right hand is going to be used to press gently against the cartilage of the nose, closing off first the right nostril with the thumb and then the left nostril with the ring finger.

The Breath

1. Close the eyes and mouth, breathing only through the nose.
2. Block off the right nostril using your thumb; exhale through the left nostril. This dispels any unwanted air from the body.
3. Inhale through the left nostril for two counts.
4. Close off the left nostril (both nostrils are closed at this point) and hold for eight counts. These are not seconds but counts – for example, 'One Om, two Om, three Om ...'
5. Release the right nostril and exhale for four counts.
6. Inhale through the right nostril for two counts.
7. Close off the right nostril (again both nostrils are closed) and hold for eight counts.
8. Release the left nostril and exhale for four counts.
9. This is one round. Repeat this for three rounds.

Ratio: inhale two, hold eight, exhale four

The outlined practice is for beginners. As time progresses or if you are a more advanced student, Anuloma Viloma can be undertaken for a ratio of inhale four, hold sixteen, exhale eight for three complete rounds.

As a practitioner becomes more familiar with the practice, the use of Bhandas can be introduced and incorporated. The three important and most commonly mentioned Bandhas are Jalandhara, Uddiyana, and Mooladhara.

Contraindications

Do not practice this if one of your nostrils is blocked.

Opening Poses

Cobbler Pose (Baddha Konasana)

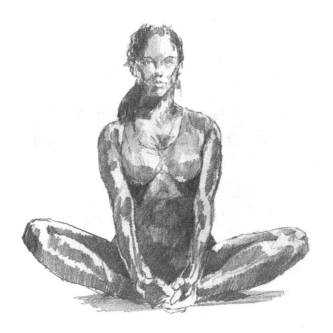

Cobbler Pose (Baddha Konasana)

1. Sit on your mat on the floor on your sitting bones with a straight back.
2. Bend the legs and bring the soles of your feet together in front of you, drawing the heels towards the pubic bone.
3. Allow the hips to open and the knees to fall to the sides, bringing them as close to the floor as your body will allow.
4. The soles of the feet can gradually be worked on so that they turn up towards the ceiling. The more these turn up towards the ceiling, the more open the hips become.
5. Sit here for approximately one minute, consciously working on and opening the hips.
6. Maintain a straight back at all times.
7. Continue to breathe deeply, letting go of any tension.

Precautions

Be cautious if you have hip or knee issues.

Contraindications

Do not sit in this pose if you have had a recent knee or hip operation. Ensure that you get clearance from your doctor before carrying out the posture.

Benefits

The posture opens the hips, particularly during pregnancy, because it stretches the pelvic floor.

Connection Number

These numbers indicate which postures are combined together to create a sexual connection and these can be seen in section three of this book. They are in numerical order from #1 through to #23.

To be used in sexual position #11 and #18.

Pigeon Pose (Kapotasana)

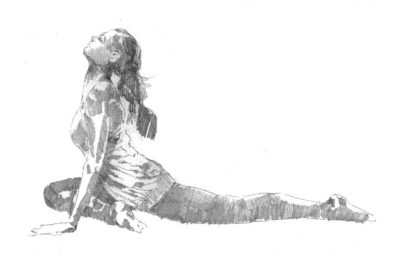

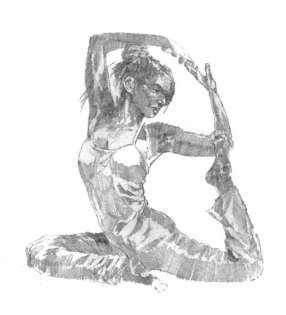

Pigeon Pose (Kapotasana)

1. Come onto all fours on your mat.
2. Bend your right knee and bring it up between your hands; place it on the floor.
3. The lower leg and foot are resting flat on the floor, and the toes point back towards you.
4. The opposing leg is straight out behind you with the toes pointing away. Again, the foot rests flat on the floor.
5. The hands and arms provide support to the upper body and torso.
6. The heel of the front foot lies in line with the pubic bone so that as the hips lower, the area of the pubic bone rests down, if comfortable, onto the heel of the foot of the bent leg. This may be an uncomfortable position for men, so adjust the body accordingly.
7. The arms are still holding the upper body up, and the palms of the hands are working into the ground. Remain here if you want to achieve the easier option.
8. For a more advanced pose; bend the back leg at the knee, lifting the foot so that the sole of the foot is facing the ceiling. The left hand wraps around the ankle and pulls the left foot in towards the buttocks. Do not strain or twist the knee, and be cautious of the back. Do not overarch or strain. The aim is for the foot to eventually nestle into the crook of the arm at the elbow. The hands join together as the body turns out to face the left side.
9. Hold this position for a few seconds, taking deep breaths.
10. To come out of the pose if fully accomplished; release the hands bringing them back to either side of the front knee, the torso turns to face forward whilst lowering the back leg to the floor.
11. To continue, swap the position of the legs; take the right leg back so it is lying flat and bring the left knee forward so it is situated between the hands and repeat the operation to the opposing side.
12. When finished, lengthen out both legs behind you so that they are flat on the floor and push back into extended swan pose and relax for a few breaths.

Precautions

Be cautious if you have any issues with the hips, back, or knees. This is a somewhat awkward posture, so take overall precaution whilst attempting it. Do not get despondent – it takes practice.

Contraindications

If you have a severe knee, back, or hip injury, or if you have had recent surgery on these areas, avoid this pose. If you have any spinal problems, do not carry out this posture.

Benefits

It stretches the psoas, groin, and thigh. The chest opens, encouraging deep, rhythmic breathing. The back receives a good stretch, relieving tightness along the spine. Flexibility in the spine is improved. It is very effective at opening the hips.

Connection Number

To be used in sexual position #8.

Sequence Work and Transition Poses

Sun Salutation (Surya Namaskar)

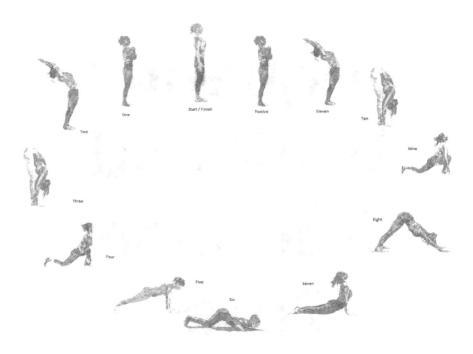

Carry out a minimum of four complete rounds to maximise the benefit.

Sun Salutation (Surya Namaskar)

In the Sun Salutation series please note that a complete round constitutes carrying out the movements on the right and left side. Always begin and work from the right side.

1. Stand in Tadasana (Mountain Pose) at the front of the mat.
2. Bring attention to the breath.
3. Put your toes and inner part of the heels together; energise the legs.
4. Draw the tailbone down towards the floor, which lifts the internal organs up towards the chest.
5. Pull the chin in gently lengthening the back of the neck.
6. Bring the arms to the sides of the body, the hands are spread and alert with the middle finger pointing downwards towards the ground.
7. Move the shoulder blades down the back keeping the shoulders away from the ears, and the chest open.

Note: Throughout the practice, use Ujjayi breath on the exhalation.

8. Inhale
9. Exhale the hands into Namaste (Prayer) position; cross over the thumbs.
10. Inhale. Reach the arms forward then up over the head into Extended Tadasana. Look up towards the fingertips.
11. Exhale forward fold into Uttanasana, hands spread at the side of the feet. Soften the knees if you need to; this will enable you to reach the floor. Look towards the knees.
12. Inhale step the right foot back, knee to floor, your chest pushing forward and open. Sink into the hips. You are in a lunge position.
13. Retain the breath whilst stepping back with the left foot into Kumbhakasana (Plank). Keep strong in the thighs, buttocks, and arms. Keep the neck long and the crown of the head pushing forward as you look down towards the ground. The heels are pushing back.

14. Exhale as the knees, chest, and chin (or forehead) move to the ground into Ashtanga Namaskar (eight point pose). Keep the hips off the floor and the bottom up.

15. Inhale into Bhujangasana (Cobra), toes lying flat, and ensure that the heels are rolled out and not touching. Keep the shoulders away from the ears. Release the buttocks whilst pushing the hands into the mat. Draw the stomach up towards the chest whilst drawing the tailbone down towards the floor.

16. Exhale into Adho Mukha Svanasana (Downward Facing Dog). Keep the fingers spread; ensure that the hands are in line with the shoulders. The inner elbow faces forward. Keep the neck (and head) in line with the upper arms. Draw the heels down towards the floor whilst the tailbone lifts towards the sky. Lengthen the ears away from the shoulders. Flatten the shoulder blades into the spine. Draw the internal organs up towards the spine (Uddiyana Bandha – for the more experienced students)

17. From round 3, when in Downward Facing Dog, hold for five breaths. This allows a deeper level of working whilst in the pose and allows you to make any necessary adjustments.

18. Inhale and step the right foot forward between the hands, the left knee is to be placed on the floor, your chest pushing forward and open; sink into the hips. You are in a lunge position.

19. Exhale bringing the left foot through to meet the right foot and forward fold, hands on the floor with the fingers spread at the side of the feet. Look towards the knees.

20. Inhale and reach the arms out to the sides of the body, lifting them up over the head. Put your hands together in prayer position, arch the back slightly clenching the buttocks to protect the back, and look towards the fingertips. Do not let the head drop beyond the arms.

21. Exhale and lower the arms down, bringing the hands into prayer pose at the heart centre.

22. Repeat on the opposite side.

Precautions

Be cautious if you have hip or knee issues.

Contraindications:

Be careful with high blood pressure if it's not under the control of the doctor. Do not retain the breath at any stage if you suffer from high blood pressure, have a hernia, have acute back conditions, are pregnant, or have heart disease or a weak heart.

Benefits

This sequence balances the endocrine, circulatory, and digestive systems. It influences the pineal gland and hypothalamus. It also encourages deep, rhythmic breathing and removes toxins from the body. It oxygenates the blood to the brain and tones the muscles.

Connection Number

To be used in foreplay #3 and #4 (mountain) and sexual positions #9 and #14 (mountain), #19 (forward bend and mountain pose from the sequence), and #23 (mountain).

Downward Facing Dog Pose (Adho Mukha Svanasana)

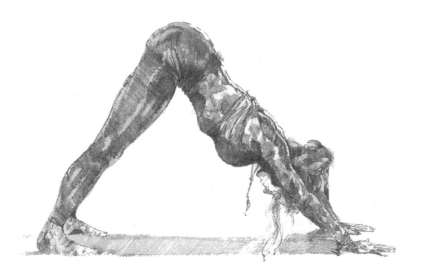

Downward Facing Dog Pose (Adho Mukha Svanasana)

1. Begin in mountain pose.
2. Inhale as you take the arms up over head allowing the palms of the hands to touch. Exhale and fold forward placing the hands either side of the feet.
3. Inhale and then exhale as you step back with the right foot followed by the left foot. These are to be placed approximately hip width apart so that the feet, hips, shoulders and hands are in line. The hips are lifting up; directing the tailbone towards the ceiling so that the body creates a triangular shape.
4. Keep breathing.
5. The heels are moving down towards the ground, the hamstrings are stretching, the palms are pushing into the floor, the head is hanging down, and the abdomen is relaxed.
6. Hold for three to five breaths.
7. To come out of the posture, look forward to between the hands. As you Inhale, lift the right leg through and place the foot between the hands, closely followed by the left leg, bringing both feet together. Exhale as you fold into a forward bend.
8. Inhale as you come up, opening and lifting the arms over head bringing the hands together in prayer. Exhale, lowering the hands to the heart centre.
9. Repeat on the opposing side.

Variations

When in Downward Facing Dog you can deepen this pose further by raising first the right leg straight out behind you up into the air without straining, hold for two to three breaths and then lower and repeat with the left leg.

Precautions

Be cautious if you have any back aches or stiffness. If you suffer with high blood pressure, then do not hold the head lower than the heart for too long.

Contraindications

If you have acute back conditions, refrain from participating in this pose. Refrain if you have a hernia, a weak heart, if you have had a stroke, or if you are pregnant (unless the knees are dropped).

Benefits

It strengthens the circulatory and nervous system. It influences the pineal gland and hypothalamus and encourages deep, rhythmic breathing. It dispels toxins from the body and oxygenates the blood. It also tones the muscles in the arms and legs. It provides mental clarity and focus.

Connection Number

To be used in sexual position #16 (variation pose).

Plank Pose (Kumbhakasana)

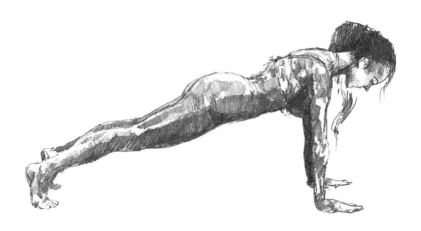

Plank Pose (Kumbhakasana)

1. Stand at the front of the mat in mountain pose.
2. Inhale.
3. Exhale hands at the heart centre in prayer position.
4. Inhale and push the hands up above the head, lengthening the arms as you look forward. Do not take the arms back further than the head.
5. Exhale folding forward placing the hands either side of the feet.
6. Inhale and exhale as you step the right foot and then the left foot back, or jump back with both legs simultaneously so that you are low and parallel to the ground.
7. Keep breathing deeply.
8. Ensure that the hands are spread.
9. The shoulders are over the wrists, and the arms are straight.
10. Keep the length in the spine. The eyes are looking down just a few inches in front of the fingertips. The head is not up, cricking the neck. The spine is elongated in one straight line.
11. Do not let the hips drop, and do not lift them; they remain neutral. You will feel that the abdominal muscles engage in the correct position.
12. Feet are together with the toes tucked under and the heels pushing away.
13. The legs are together with the thigh muscles drawing up with slight tension.
14. The buttocks are active.
15. Lengthen the spine from the crown of the head to the heels.
16. Hold for a few breaths or as long as is comfortable. This pose is often used as a transitional position so from here you would move into another posture.

Precautions

Do not retain the breath if you have high blood pressure. Be careful not to over strain the hands, wrists, arms and toes. Be careful not to strain the abdomen or spine.

Contraindications

Do not carry out this pose if you have carpal tunnel syndrome or are intoxicated. If you have had a recent operation or abdominal surgery, have severe back or shoulder problems, avoid carrying out this pose. Always seek medical advice.

Benefits

It strengthens the arms, wrists and spine. It tones the abdomen, back, and shoulders. It eliminates toxins from the body and lengthens the spine.

Connection Number:

To be used in sexual positions #17 and #18.

Standing
Poses

Crescent Moon Pose (Anjaneyasana)

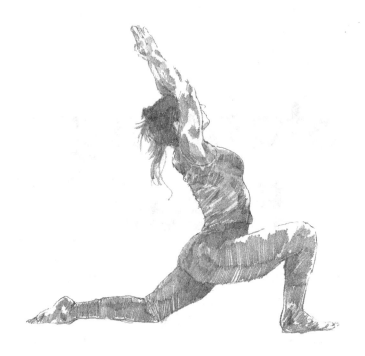

Crescent Moon Pose (Anjaneyasana)

1. Stand in mountain pose.
2. Inhale and take the arms up so that the palms of the hands touch overhead. Exhale into forward fold, positioning the hands at the side of the feet. Bend the knees if you need to.
3. Inhale, and then as you exhale, step the right foot back, placing the lower leg along the floor with the toes pointing away from you; the left leg is bent at the knee. You will be in a lunge position.
4. Place the hands together in prayer at the heart centre.
5. As you Inhale, push the hands out in front of you and up moving the upper body from the hips forward in one continuous, flowing movement. As you exhale, arch backwards, taking the arms over head and back as far as is comfortable. Do not let the head drop further back than the arms.
6. Continue to breathe.
7. Keep pushing forward through the hips; bring some tension into the buttocks to protect the back; do not strain the back.
8. The body creates a beautiful arch, the crescent moon. This is to be carried out on both sides of the body. When you are ready, slowly come out of the arch bringing the arms down and placing the hands on either side of the front foot.
9. Inhale and step the back foot forward between the hands. Exhale, take the opposing foot back, and repeat on the other side.

Precautions

Take caution with regards to the knees and back.

Contraindications

Do not practice if you suffer with acute back problems. Do not practice this pose if you have had any recent injuries or operations to the knees.

Benefits

This pose develops a good sense of balance over a period of time. It gives a wonderful stretch along the front of the body, and it encourages deep breathing.

Connection Number

To be used in foreplay position #5.

Wide Leg Standing Forward Bend Pose (Prasarita Padottanasana)

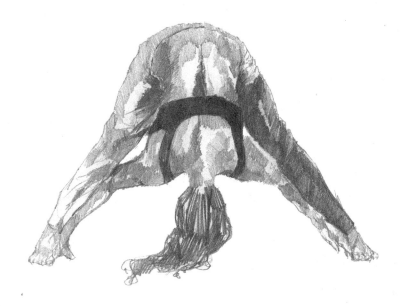

Wide Leg Standing Forward Bend Pose
(Prasarita Padottanasana)

1. Stand with the legs wide apart and the feet parallel. The wider the feet, the easier the stretch, but work with what feels the most comfortable for you.
2. Place the hands on the hips* and Inhale, opening across the chest.
3. As you exhale, hinge forward from the hips, bending down slowly keeping the spine long and moving the head towards the ground.
4. Ensure that the back remains flat and do not over stretch.
5. Continue to breathe.
6. Place the palms of the hands flat on the floor and if possible, bend the elbows bringing the top of the head even closer to the ground. Continue to work with the breath.
7. Feel energy rising up through the legs and down through the spine.
8. Continue to feel the posture working at all times.
9. Remain in the position for approximately two to three breaths.
10. To come out of the posture, place the hands back on the hips, bend the knees, and slowly lift the upper body in the reverse manner in which you lowered it. Be careful to not do this too quickly, as you may go dizzy.
11. Release the posture and move the legs back together.

*Alternative arm positions:

Clasp the hands behind the back and straighten the arms.
Lift the arms out and up behind the body as you lower forward.

Place the hands in prayer position behind the back, up towards the shoulder blades. Lower into the position as previously stated. If you are unable to achieve prayer position, then hold onto the elbows behind the back.

Using the first two fingers and the thumb of each hand as you lower forward, grasp the big toe on each foot, right hand to right foot, left hand to left foot.

Precautions

Be cautious if you have any back or hip issues not listed below. If you have high blood pressure, keep the head above the heart level; therefore only bend forward to a ninety-degree angle.

Contraindications

This should not be practised by those who have a slipped disc or sciatica. If you have high blood pressure, heart conditions, inflammation within the ear, any eye disorders, defective thyroid or pituitary glands, severe asthma, a cold or sinusitis, arteriosclerosis, cerebral or other thrombosis, vertigo, or blood issues, you should not carry out this pose.

Benefits

In the case of low blood pressure, this posture may help. It balances the nervous system and brings a rich supply of blood to the brain.

Triangle Pose (Trikonasana)

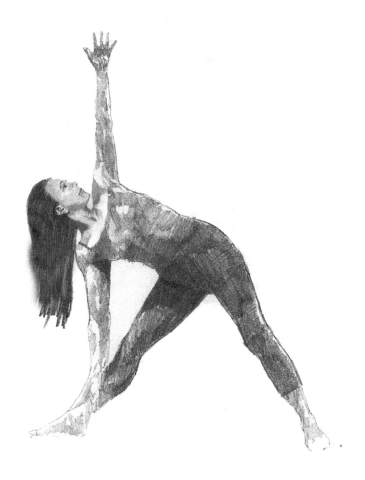

Triangle Pose (Trikonasana)

1. Stand on the mat with the legs apart. The feet are approximately five of your foot lengths away from each other. This can be jumped or stepped into.
2. Ensure that the feet are parallel and that the toes are pointing forward.
3. Inhale as you lift the arms up, bringing the hands together in prayer overhead. Exhale as you lower them to shoulder height. The arms are outstretched.
4. Drop the shoulders down the back; do not hunch the shoulders up around the ears.
5. Inhale and then exhale as you raise the right foot onto the heel and turn it out ninety degrees before lowering the foot back down again. This will be classed as the front leg.
6. Inhale and turn the left foot in slightly, approximately fifteen degrees, and exhale. This is classed as the back foot.
7. Keep breathing. Check to ensure that the heels are in line. (Beginners can line up the heels with the back of the mat, if that helps.)
8. Turn the head to look over the right hand.
9. Inhale and extend the right hand forward, reaching out over the front leg.
10. Exhale and lower the hand to the shin, ankle or floor. Wherever is the most comfortable without compromising the rest of the posture.
11. Remain looking down at the foot.
12. Breathe.
13. Push the hips forward slightly and tighten the buttocks whilst lengthening the upper body and lifting the ribs. Imagine you are flattening the back of your body against a wall whilst being supported by its rigidity.
14. Open the chest and draw the shoulder blades together as you lengthen the left arm up overhead. Spread the fingers. The arms are in one continuous line from the right (lower) hand through the shoulders and up to the left hand.

15. If comfortable and balanced, inhale and exhale as you rotate the head to look up at the top hand.
16. Lift the thigh muscles, gently locking the kneecaps but not overstraining. Push against the imaginary wall. The body should be aligned over the knee. *Do not lean forward or back.* Tuck the chin in towards the shoulder slightly.
17. Hold for three to five breaths.
18. To come out of the posture, it is important if you have rotated the head that you turn the head first to look down at the front foot / towards the floor, before you move any other part of the body.
19. Lift, using the force of the upper arm and bring yourself to an upright position with both of the arms resting outstretched at shoulder height, turn the head so that you are looking straight ahead and rotate the feet so that they are parallel once more. Repeat the process on the left side.

Precautions

If you suffer with a bad neck or dizziness, then ensure that you remain looking down towards the front foot and not up towards the hand. Carry out the pose against a wall if you do not feel stable. Use props such as blocks under the lower hand to raise the pose if you are performing this posture whilst pregnant, or rest the hands above the knee. Do not go deep into this pose whilst pregnant.

Contraindications

Do not carry out if you suffer with either high or low blood pressure, if you are intoxicated, or if you have a heart condition. If you have severe neck injuries, do not do this posture. However, ensure you consult your doctor because it may assist certain neck problems. Do not carry out if you have lower back issues or a hernia.

Benefits

This pose strengthens and stretches the hips, knees, and areas of the ankle. It helps to relieve stress, anxiety, and nervous disorders, and it works on the spinal nerves. It can tone the abdominal and reproductive organs, as well as help with digestion and circulation. It assists with flat feet, some neck issues, sciatica, and osteoporosis.

Connection

To be used in sexual position #13, for both parties.

Warrior I Pose (Virabhadrasana I)

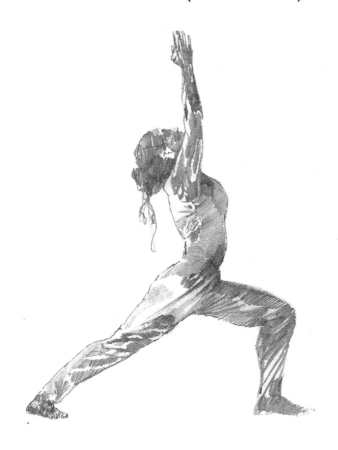

Warrior I Pose (Virabhadrasana I)

1. Stand on your mat with the feet approximately five of your own foot lengths apart. Jump or step into position.
2. Ensure that the feet are parallel and the toes are pointing forward.
3. Lift the right foot onto the heel and turn it out ninety degrees before lowering the toes so that the foot is flat on the mat once again.
4. Turn the left foot in slightly and gently press the outer edge into the floor ensuring that it does not lift whilst carrying out the posture.
5. The hips should be rotated and facing towards the front foot (the one you turned out ninety degrees).
6. At this point, check that the middle toe of the front foot is pointing forwards.
7. The front leg is bent so that the thigh is parallel to the floor. The big toe will be seen as you look past the knee joint, and the knee is over the centre of the heel, creating one line from the ankle to the knee.
8. The back leg is straight.
9. Inhale as you raise the arms up overhead. The palms of the hands come together in prayer; the fingers can be closed or spread. In either case the fingers need to be active.
10. Straighten the arms.
11. Exhale as you sink deeply into the posture and gently drop the head back, looking up towards the hands over head.
12. Hold the pose for three to five deep breaths.
13. The eyes should be looking past the fingertips.
14. The sternum should be lifted.
15. The slight spinal arch should come from the upper back and not the lower back.
16. Remain relaxed and keep the breathing rhythmic.
17. To come out of the posture, first look straight ahead. Bring the hands down to the heart centre in prayer pose. Rotate both feet so that they are parallel once again before performing it on the opposing side.

Precautions

If you have neck problems, then remain looking ahead and not upward. Be very cautious if you suffer with the ankles, knees, hips, back, or shoulders.

Contraindications

If you have had a recent ankle, knee, hip, back, or shoulder injury, or if you have had an operation, then do not perform this posture.

Benefits

This pose strengthens the legs and stretches the arms and legs, increasing flexibility. It opens the hips and chest, improving the circulatory and respiratory systems, which energises the entire body. Balance is also improved.

Connection

To be used in sexual positions #10, #15 and #16.

Twisting Pose

Half Spinal Twist Pose (Ardha Matsyendrasana)

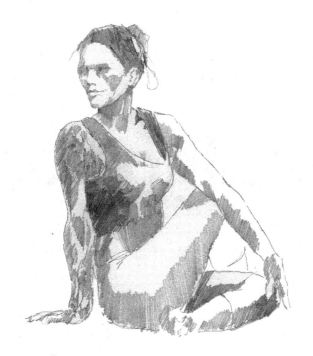

Half Spinal Twist Pose (Ardha Matsyendrasana)

1. Sit on your knees on your mat.
2. Move your weight over onto your left hip as you bring the legs out to the right side still folded.
3. The leg left stays in the lower position and is bent at the knee. The left heel sits to the outer edge of the right buttock.
4. Cross the right leg over the left leg with the right knee pointing towards the sky, and the tips of the toes of the right foot approximately in line with the left knee if possible.
5. Inhale, raise the right arm up, and sweep it behind you, resting the fingers on the floor for balance.
6. Bring the left elbow to the top of the right knee placing the thumb in line with the nose; this balances the perineum and crown.
7. Inhale and raise the left arm straight up towards the sky. Exhale as you stretch the left arm across the front of the body, placing the back of the upper left arm on the far side of the outer edge of right knee. Try to slide the left shoulder down as close to the right knee as possible. Rest the forearm of the left arm along the outer edge of the right thigh. The left hand rests on the outside of the right buttock. Keep breathing. (If this position is too difficult to achieve, then wrap the left arm around the right knee and rest the crook of the left elbow around the front of the right knee.)
8. Inhale as you breathe into the chest; lengthen the spine and rotate to the right. Lead with the shoulder followed by the chin, keeping the spine fully in line. The shoulders should be level; ensure you remain on the sitting bones. Elongate the back of the neck keeping the chin slightly tucked in. Do not lean to the side.
9. Close the eyes to maintain the focus.
10. Continue to try to breathe into the belly even though it may feel restricted as this stimulates the eliminative organs.
11. Stay for a minimum of eight breaths. Take deep Inhalations, and as you exhale, twist more to the right. The twist comes from the waist and not the top of the back or shoulders.

12. To come out of the pose, inhale, and as you exhale rotate the head so that you are looking forward, followed by the upper body. Release the arms and legs and prepare to repeat on the other side, sitting on the right buttock.

Precautions

Be cautious if you have any neck or back issues. This position can be quite strong on the internal organs. Be very cautious if you are menstruating, because it can be a powerful abdominal twist.

Contraindications

Do not practice this particular method during pregnancy. If you suffer from a hernia, ulcers, or hyperthyroidism, then you should seek expert advice. Do not practice if you have severe spinal problems or a slipped disc, although those with a mild slip disc may benefit from this pose. It is advised that you seek medical advice. Do not carry out if you have a crumbling lumbar or lower back injury.

Benefits

It massages the eliminative organs, assisting the body in getting rid of waste and stopping it building up in the colon. It tones the abdomen and releases pain, stiffness, and tension in the spine, as well as between the vertebrae. It can help with minor slipped disc and improves rounded shoulders. The pose stretches the muscles down the side of the body, opens the chest, and increases the oxygen supply to the lungs. It relieves stiffness in the hip joints and opens and loosens the hips. It regulates the secretion of bile and adrenalin. It releases tension in the shoulders, upper back, and neck. It improves the health of the reproductive organs and the urinary system due to increased nutrients and oxygen within the fresh blood supply targeting these areas whilst twisting. It relieves any tension built up from doing forward and backward asanas.

Balance Poses

Tree Pose (Vrksasana)

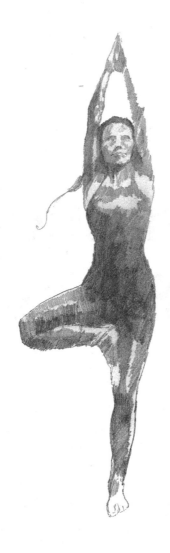

Tree Pose (Vrksasana)

1. Stand at the front of the mat in mountain pose.
2. Inhale.
3. Exhale hands to prayer pose at the heart centre.
4. Keep breathing.
5. Find a still point in front of you to focus on (not a person). Remember that when the eyes move, so does the body.
6. Calm the mind. Imagine the mind as an erratic snowstorm; watch as it calms and the snowflakes flutter down.
7. Notice the breath and watch as it relaxes.
8. Move the weight to the left leg and foot; soften the leg at the knee.
9. Lift the right leg and place the right foot onto the inner thigh of the left leg. Use the hand around the ankle to assist placing the foot. If you are unable to place the foot high up on the thigh, then place it against the opposing ankle. This is a modification. Press the sole of the foot firmly into the left thigh with the heel as high as possible towards the groin, toes pointing towards the ground. Never place the foot against the knee. The standing leg is strong but not locked. Bring focus to the foot on the floor, bringing particular attention to the contact points of the big toe, little toe, heel, and the position of the ankle. Imagine roots growing out of the foot and into the ground, giving you strength and stability in the left leg.
10. Inhale.
11. Exhale and bring the hands back to prayer at the heart centre. Ensure that the elbows are pointing out to the sides and the arms level. Lengthen the tailbone towards the ground and feel the abdomen engage.
12. Hold for five breaths in tree pose.
13. To continue further - Cross the thumbs.
14. Inhale and push the arms forward and up over the head. Exhale as you squeeze the arms slightly in line with the ears.
15. Inhale.
16. Exhale and bend the elbows; drop the hands back behind the head. Keep breathing. Ensure that the tailbone continues to feel

lengthened and abdominals are engaged. Feel the chest opening. Hold for two further breaths

17. Once complete, inhale and raise the arms back up over head
18. Exhale and hold for three further breaths.
19. To come out of the posture, bring the hands back down to the heart centre and release the bent leg. Balance out the weight with both feet on the floor.
20. Repeat on the other side.

Precautions

If you struggle to achieve this pose due to balancing issues, use a wall or the rear of a high-backed chair for support. If it is uncomfortable bringing the hands together overhead in prayer, then open the arms, place the first finger and thumb together with the rest of the fingers outstretched in chin mudra, and create blossoming tree.

Contraindications

If you have had a recent knee operation or leg injury, then avoid this pose. If you suffer with vertigo, do not carry out this pose.

Benefits

It strengthens the leg muscles and improves concentration and focus. It tones the abdomen and gives the chest a large open area to ensure deep breathing when the arms are overhead, which improves oxygenation in the blood. It develops and strengthens the nervous system.

Connection Number:

To be used in foreplay position #3.

Extended Hand to Big Toe Pose (Utthita Hasta Padangusthasana)

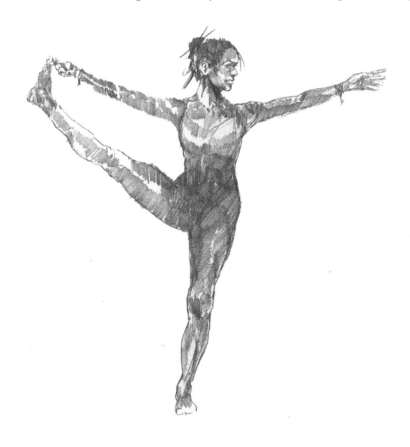

Extended Hand to Big Toe Pose (Utthita Hasta Padangusthasana)

1. Stand at the front of the mat in mountain pose.
2. Inhale.
3. Exhale hands to prayer pose at the heart centre.
4. Keep breathing.
5. Find a still point in front of you to focus on (not a person). Remember that when the eyes move, so does the body.
6. Calm the mind.
7. Notice the breath and see how it relaxes.
8. Move the weight to the left leg and foot; soften the leg.
9. Place the left hand on the left hip. Once in position, raise the left arm out and up in the air.
10. Inhale as you bend the right leg, bringing the knee up towards the chest and grasping hold of the big right toe using the first two fingers and thumb of the right hand. The arm and hand moves down on the inside of the leg.
11. Exhale as you extend the right leg out in front of you whilst still holding onto the toe, bringing it up as high as is comfortable for you. Bend the knee if you need to.
12. The knee of the supporting leg is relaxed and not locked, and the buttocks are slightly tilting under.
13. Keep breathing. Be calm and steady in the pose. Hold for a few breaths.
14. To come out of the pose, release the big toe, bring the right knee into the chest, and lower the leg down. The hands come back to prayer pose at the heart centre.
15. Repeat on the opposite side.

Precautions

If you struggle to achieve this pose due to balancing issues, use a wall or the rear of a high-backed chair for support.

Contraindications

If you have had a recent knee operation or leg injury, then avoid this pose. If you suffer with vertigo, do not carry out this pose. Do not do if you have sciatica or hip complaints.

Benefits

It improves the level of focus and concentration whilst balancing and coordinating the muscles with the nervous system. The hips and leg muscles are strengthened and toned.

Connection Number

To be used in foreplay position #6 and sexual position #23.

Lord Shiva's Pose or Dancer Pose (Natarajasana)

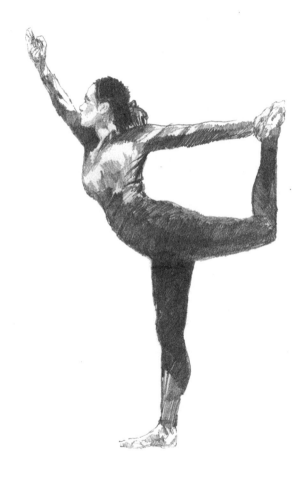

Lord Shiva's Pose or Dancer Pose (Natarajasana)

1. Stand in mountain pose.
2. Move the feet to hip width apart.
3. Change your weight slightly so that more of the weight is on the left leg in preparation.
4. Draw the muscles of the leg up to take pressure off the knee.
5. Raise the left arm straight up so that the fingers point towards the ceiling and the arm is along the side of the head, close to the ear.
6. Focus on a spot in front of you to assist with balance.
7. Bend the right leg behind you and hold onto the foot, ankle, or calf with the right hand, whichever is the most comfortable.
8. Slowly begin to lower the torso in a forward motion. The left arm will also move forward with the upper body, and as this occurs, simultaneously raise the right leg out behind you, still holding onto it. The sole of the right foot should be facing up towards the ceiling.
9. Hold for two to three breaths.
10. To come out of the pose simply reverse the action. Slowly lift the torso, the arm will automatically move at the same time, whilst simultaneously lowering the leg. You will finish upright. However, the leg will still be bent at the knee and the arm in the air. Lower these to come back to the starting position of mountain pose.
11. Repeat on the opposite side. Take your time with the posture.

Precautions

Be cautious if you have any back issues. If you suffer with balance, then use either the back of a stable chair or a wall to hold for support.

Contraindications

Do not carry out this posture if you have severe back issues, or if you have had surgery or a recent injury to the knees or ankles.

Benefits

This asana is balancing to the nervous system. It assists in developing and enhancing concentration, and it increases suppleness in the legs.

Connection Number

To be used in sexual position #9.

Crow Pose (Khakasana)

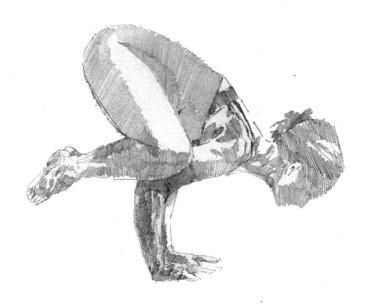

Crow Pose (Khakasana)

1. Come down to the mat in a squatting position, balancing on your toes. The heels are together, and the knees are apart.
2. The arms are lengthened with the back of the hands resting against the inner knees. The hands are in chin mudra, which means that the tip of the first finger and thumb rest together as the remaining three fingers are outstretched.
3. Push your hands back gently against the knees.
4. Straighten the back.
5. Begin to focus the eyes on a non-moving spot a few feet in front of you.
6. Notice your breathing.
7. Allow the mind to become peaceful before the next stage.
8. Release the hands and stretch the arms out in front of you. Lower the hands and place the palms flat on the ground in front of you. The middle fingers are pointing forwards, and the rest of the fingers are spread out. The hands are placed close together with the thumbs around three inches apart.
9. Start to rock back and forth on the hands, slightly lifting your weight. At this point test your balance and the weight change.
10. Your knees will sit on the upper arm above the elbow, approximately on the tricep muscle.
11. Keep focused on the point ahead, with your chin up and your chest open.
12. Try this a few times.
13. When you feel ready to take the feet off the floor for longer, begin by lifting just one foot and then the other.
14. The use of the arms here is imperative in keeping the chest open and powerful. The chest needs to be filled with as much prana and oxygen as possible. It is a very powerful pose, so energy is of paramount importance.
15. Remember to continue to keep breathing
16. Inhale slowly as you take the weight of the body onto the upper arms and hands.

17. Bring the big toes together.
18. Keep the fingers spread and pushing into the mat as you exhale.
19. Feel the strength in your arms as you squeeze the knees against the upper arm.
20. Keep the head up and look forward. Feel stabilised and steady, and keep your focus. Try to hold for two to five breaths. Enjoy the flight!

Precautions

Take great care and follow the instructions carefully. The pose is not overly difficult but is quite precise.

Contraindications

If you suffer with high blood pressure, then do not carry out this posture. Do not attempt this posture if pregnant, if you have heart problems or cerebral thrombosis, or if you are intoxicated.

Benefits

The pose strengthens the arms and wrists. It improves concentration and physical balance, and it strengthens the nervous system.

Connection Number

To be used in foreplay position #1.

Boat Pose (Navasana)

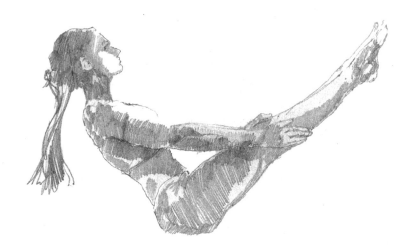

Boat Pose (Navasana)

1. Sit on your mat on your bottom.
2. Rest on the sitting bones with the legs straight out in front of you and the back straight.
3. Point the toes.
4. Rest your hands behind you for stability. Place them close to the body with the fingers pointing in towards your back.
5. Now that you are stable, gently lean back into the hands whilst simultaneously bending the knees and bringing them towards the torso.
6. Once you feel stable on the sitting bones, carefully lengthen the legs so that they are raised out in front of you. Keep pointing the toes. Do not expect to straighten the legs immediately; it is perfectly acceptable to have the knees bent.
7. Draw in the core muscles of the stomach and keep the chest lifted and open. The head is lifted and you look straight ahead.
8. Keep taking steady, full breaths.
9. When you feel confident and steady, bring the arms to the front of the body and stretch them out in front of you. Turn the palms of the hands in towards the body, keeping the fingers lengthened and together, the thumb points up towards the sky. The body creates a V shape.
10. Complete three rounds and hold each round for five breaths.

Easier Option

If you do not feel comfortable bringing the arms out in front of you, then allow them to remain supporting you in their original position resting on the floor behind you. The core muscles will still be working.

Precaution

Be cautious if you have any lower back issues.

Contraindications

Do not carry out if you have severe spinal issues, particularly in the lower back. If you have had an injury or recent operation to the abdomen area, do not attempt this posture. If you have high blood pressure, heart issues, a slipped disc, or sciatica, do not carry out this pose.

Benefits

It helps to strengthen and tone abdominal muscles and organs whilst strengthening the back and helping with realignment of the spine. It assists with developing focus, coordination, and concentration. It helps to eliminate waste from the intestine, alleviating constipation. It aids the parasympathetic and sympathetic elements of the nervous system.

Connection Number

To be used in foreplay position #2 and sexual position #21 (arms leaning back).

Inversion Poses

Shoulder Stand Pose (Sarvangasana)

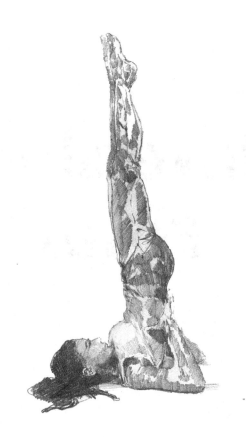

Shoulder Stand Pose (Sarvangasana)

1. Lie on your back on the floor on your mat with the arms straight down at the side of the body, palms facing down.
2. Align the body and tuck in the chin to protect the neck.
3. Using the body's momentum, bend the knees towards the chest whilst simultaneously pushing the palms into the ground. Use the abdominal muscles to send energy through the legs, pushing the soles of the feet up towards the ceiling. The hips effectively roll up and over the shoulders so that the body in is line.
4. The elbows are bent, and therefore the tops of the arms remain resting on the floor whilst the remainder of the arm is vertical. The hands should clasp around the hips, providing support for the back.
5. The neck is elongated, with the chin tucked in. Ensure that you keep breathing and keep lifting up through the legs, drawing strength from the core. The feet are flexed, meaning that the soles are parallel with the ceiling.
6. Relax into the position and hold for at least thirty seconds, if possible. Two minutes is preferable because this is when inverted postures begin to work efficiently and alter the blood flow to the brain.
7. To come out of the posture, bend the knees towards the forehead, release the arms and lower the legs slowly, rolling back down to the mat uncurling the spine using the abdominal muscles for control.
8. Relax for a moment when you come out of the pose.

Precautions

Be cautious if you have any neck, shoulder or spine issues.

Contraindications

If you have high blood pressure, glaucoma, or other eye disorders including detached retina, then do not carry out this pose. If you have spinal injuries, a slipped disc or vertebral fusion, or neck injuries such as whiplash or severe tightness in the neck through injury, do not attempt this posture. If you have had recent surgery or have a heart condition, if you are menstruating, or if you have toothache or kyphosis, remove this pose out of your practice session.

Benefits

It stimulates the endocrine, nervous, and lymphatic systems. It strengthens the arms, shoulders, neck, back, and abdominal muscles. It repositions vital internal organs, which assists in aligning the spine. It improves the circulatory system and relieves varicose veins.

Connection Number

To be used in foreplay position #4 and sexual position #10.

Plough Pose (Halasana)

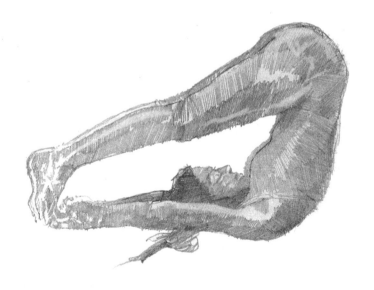

Plough Pose (Halasana)

It is advisable and easier to go into this position from the shoulder stand.

If you are aware that your feet will not touch the ground when the legs are over your head then make the necessary preparations before going into the posture. Place a folded blanket, a pillow, or a block where the toes are going to end up once you are in position.

1. Lie down on your mat with the legs extended and the arms down by your sides, with the palms of the hands facing downward.
2. Inhale and gradually raise both of the legs up towards the ceiling as if going into shoulder stand, whilst simultaneously pushing the palms of the hands into the floor.
    Once the legs are up in the air, use your hands to support the lower back. As you exhale, lower the feet over the head towards the floor. Keep breathing. It is important to have full control of this posture so that you do not damage your spine. Keep the back lengthened and move in a controlled manner. The legs remain straight if possible. The toes touch the floor behind your head, giving you the opportunity to press the toes into the floor, and push the heels away. If it is not possible for the toes to touch the floor, do not strain. Bend the knees as this may help, or carry out the above preparation.
3. Keep the neck long and the chin tucked in, and remember to breathe. Hold for around thirty seconds.
4. To come out of the pose, use the arms as brakes, placing them flat on your mat with the palms of the hands pushing into the floor. Come out of the posture in a controlled manner, taking care not to damage the spine. Use the abdominal muscles as you slowly unfold the body releasing it vertebrae by vertebrae back down to the mat. Finally lower the legs once the spine is comfortably on the ground.
5. Relax in corpse pose.

Different leg movements can be attempted once you feel confident and strong in the posture.

Option one:
Open the legs so that they are wide apart and bring the toes to touch the floor pushing the heels away

Option two:
Bend the knees to the ears and rest the lower part of the leg flat along the floor with the toes flattened out

Precautions

Be cautious if you have any neck, shoulder or back issues.

Contraindications and Benefits

See the shoulder stand advisory notes.

Connection Number

To be used in sexual position #10 (alternative).

Inversion Counter Pose

Fish Pose (Matsyasana)

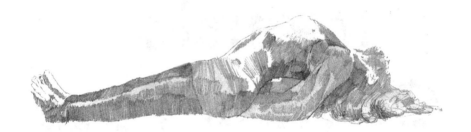

Fish Pose (Matsyasana)

1. Lie on your back on your mat.
2. Remember to keep breathing throughout the following.
3. Bend the knees and place the feet on the mat hip width apart.
4. Lift the hips high up.
5. Place the hands underneath you, locking the thumbs together by crossing them over.
6. Lengthen the arms whilst the thumbs are still crossed, pushing the hands down the mat towards your feet and the front of the mat.
7. The elbows will lie underneath the rib area.
8. Lower the body onto the arms and straighten out the legs, keeping them together.
9. The feet are flexed, and the toes are pulling back towards the head.
10. Move the body gently to the left and then the right, rolling the shoulders underneath the body and keeping the arms long. You may feel a slight stretch across the chest and it opening up enabling you to take in more air.
11. Separate the thumbs at this stage, lying them flat on the floor with the palms down. Spread the hands.
12. Lift the chest as you gently push the hands and forearms into the floor. The elbows are bent, and the back arches.
13. The head carefully hangs backwards; this is supported by the shoulder girdle.
14. Rest the top of the head on the floor if possible, taking the gaze behind you
15. The head should only rest lightly on the floor (or this will decrease the blood supply to the brain). Take two to three breaths provided you are comfortable.
16. Try to relax in the pose.
17. To come out of the posture, release and slowly lower the head first, followed by lowering the chest down. Finally move the arms from underneath the body by gradually rolling from side to side again, releasing first the left then the right.

Precautions

Be cautious if you have any neck or back issues. Those suffering with low blood pressure must not tilt the head backwards and must remain looking ahead.

Contraindications

Do not practice this posture if you have a hernia. Do not drop the head back if you have severe neck issues or injuries such as whiplash. If you have severe back problems, do not attempt this posture. Do not practice this pose if you are pregnant, have peptic ulcer, have heart problems, or suffer with arthritis within the hands, wrists, and elbows.

Benefits

This posture opens the chest to encourage deep and rhythmic breathing. It can aid asthma sufferers and those with bronchitis by encouraging deep respiration. It tones and stretches the abdominal organs and intestines. It alleviates backache and cervical spondylitis. It regulates the thyroid gland as well as the thymus gland, boosting the immune system. The circulation within the body is stimulated to the pelvic organs, and it helps to remove and prevent disorders to the reproductive system.

Backward Bend Poses

Bridge Pose (Setu Bandhasana Sarvangasana)

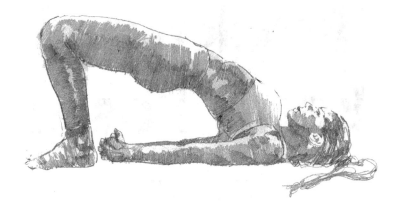

Bridge Pose (Setu Bandhasana Sarvangasana)

1. Lay down on the mat.
2. Bend the knees and bring the heels in close to your buttocks. Then place your feet flat on the floor approximately hip width apart. The feet will help to drive the posture.
3. The arms will remain flat on the floor with the palms facing down whilst you get into position. They will be used to help maintain the body's lift. During the accomplishment of the pose, slightly push the arms into the ground as this will give assistance to the elevation process.
4. Inhale, and as you exhale, lift the hips up off the floor, pushing them towards the ceiling. Squeeze the buttocks gently, which will help to maintain the lift.

   (To enhance and deepen the posture further, interlace the fingers together and roll the shoulders underneath the body starting with the right then left. This will elevate the chest opening it to increase your breath intake. If this is too difficult remain in position as outlined in point 3 with the arms flat on the floor.)
5. Tuck in the chin, elongating the neck.
6. Hold the position for approximately thirty seconds to a minute, remembering to breathe deeply and rhythmically throughout. You can close the eyes if you wish and focus.
7. To come out of the posture, slowly release the arms if you have interlaced the hands beneath the back by placing them flat on the floor at the side of the body before lowering the hips down to the mat and straightening the legs.
8. Relax and take a breath.

Precautions

Be cautious if you have any neck or back issues. Pressure can be placed upon the knees and ankles, so ensure you are careful if you have problems with these areas.

Contraindications

If you suffer with high blood pressure, then do not carry out this pose if it is not under control by a doctor; get health clearance first. If you have had a recent operation, do not carry out the pose. If you have an abdominal hernia or ulcers, do not do this pose. If you are pregnant, particularly in the latter stages, then avoid unless expertly advised.

Benefits

This pose is a good counterpose to forward bending movements, and it alleviates spinal pressure. It assists in realigning the spine, assists in eliminating rounded shoulders, and gives relief to backache. It stretches the colon and massages the abdominal organs, which improves digestion. It can help women because it tones the reproductive organs.

Connection Number

To be used in sexual position #12.

Wheel Pose (Chakrasana)

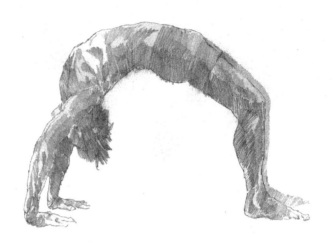

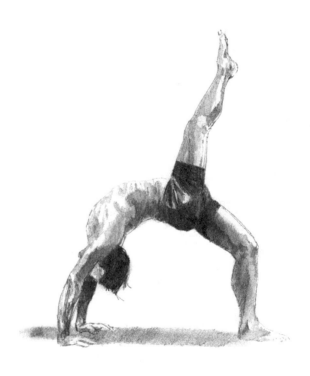

Wheel Pose (Chakrasana)

This position is strong, so be cautious. You should only attempt this posture if you have a good regular yoga practice.

1. Lie down on your back on the mat.
2. Bend the knees and place the feet flat on the floor approximately hip width apart. Slide the heels in close to the bottom. Ensure that the knees do not splay out.
3. Bend the elbows and bring the palms of the hands up and over the top of the shoulders, placing them flat on the floor at shoulder width. The fingers point down towards the shoulders and elbows point up to the sky. Do not allow the elbows to splay out.
4. The palms of the hands and soles of the feet are going to be used as the contact points on the floor. As you lift, push into the hands and feet whilst moving the body up off the ground.
5. Raise the pelvis up towards the ceiling. The buttocks are taut, the arms and legs are strong, and the neck is relaxed as the head drops backwards so that your eyes are looking behind you.
6. Continue to breathe deeply.
7. As already stated, this is a very strong posture, and eventually after plenty of practice that will inevitably build strength, the pose can be held for a number of breaths. Initially be content with achieving the posture, and allow progress to be slow but powerful. Do not strain in the posture and lower down as soon as you are ready.
8. Take your time when coming out of the posture; ensure that when you release the pose, it is carried out in a controlled manner. Lower the body down gently to the floor, taking care not to damage the neck.
9. Release the hands and feet.
10. Rotate the wrists and ankles a couple of times to release any tension in these areas.
11. Rest for a couple of breaths.

Precautions

Be cautious if you have any neck or back issues. Do not over strain the wrists.

Contraindications

This pose should not be practiced if you are pregnant, if you have weak wrists, have severe back conditions, heart problems, high or low blood pressure, glaucoma or if you have any type of illness, including severe tiredness or a headache. If you have had recent abdominal surgery or an operation or treatment of any kind refrain from doing this pose.

Benefits

This pose is particularly beneficial to the respiratory, digestive, cardiovascular, endocrine, and nervous systems. It influences hormonal secretion and can help with gynaecological disorders.

Connection Number

To be used in sexual position #14.

Cobra Pose (Bhujangasana)

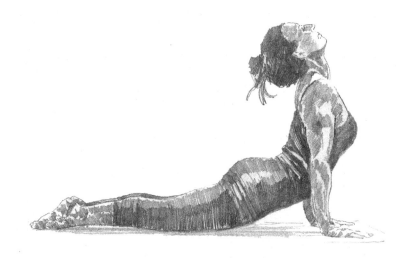

Cobra Pose (Bhujangasana)

1. Lie face down on the mat with your forehead resting on the floor.
2. Place the palms of your hands on the floor with the fingertips approximately in line with the top of the shoulders.
3. Elbows are bent and in the air, pointing behind you but close to the sides of the upper body.
4. Bring the legs together, ensuring that the heels are turned out to take pressure off the sciatic nerve.
5. Keep the legs active during the posture.
6. As you inhale, slowly stroke the floor with the nose and chin as you begin to lift, lengthening the arms and driving the head and torso forward and up. Exhale. Keep breathing rhythmically throughout.
7. Use the power of the abdominal muscles to keep strong in the lift.
8. Press the hands into the floor and keep the elbows tucked in.
9. Begin to arch back slowly whilst engaging the buttocks to protect the lumbar spine. Release once in position.
10. Pull the shoulders back and down.
11. Allow the spine to curve slowly and purposefully creating an arch in the back without collapsing the neck.
12. The thighs are to remain touching the floor. Imagine you are the inside of a wheel.
13. Hold for five to eight breaths if able.
14. To come out of the posture, exhale slowly as you lower back down to the floor, reversing the way in which you entered the pose.

Easier Option

An easier option is to carry out is the Sphinx pose, where the flat of the forearm remains on the floor by creating a ninety degree angle at the elbow. From the elbow to the fingertips remain on the floor rather than having a straight arm. The elbow should be placed in line with the shoulder. Lift the chest and head but without overarching.

Precautions

Be cautious if you have any neck or back issues.

Contraindications

If you have a hernia or have had recent abdominal surgery, do not attempt this posture. If you suffer with a slipped disc or have back issues, or if you have problems with the sciatic nerve that is severe, do not practice this pose.

Benefits

It strengthens the legs and stretches the hamstrings whilst increasing flexibility in the hip joints. It tones and massages the entire abdominal and pelvic region, including the liver, pancreas, spleen, kidneys, and adrenal glands. It stimulates digestion and relieves constipation. It stimulates circulation to the nerves and muscles of the back.

Connection Number

To be used in foreplay positions #2 and #7, and sexual position #21.

Camel Pose (Ustrasana)

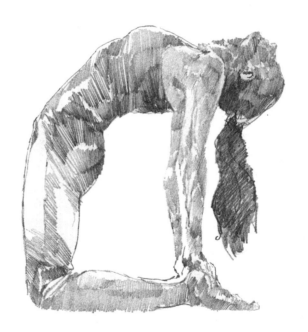

Camel Pose (Ustrasana)

This position is strong, so be cautious. You should only attempt this posture if you have a good regular yoga practice.

1. Kneel on your mat with the knees hip width apart and feet flat.
2. Place the hands on the lower back with the fingers pointing down towards the ground. Push the hips forward as if you are pushing them against a wall.
3. Lift the chest at this point as you slowly bend backwards, arching the back. As you do this, the hands slide down the buttocks, continuing down the legs and towards the ankle before grasping each of the heels. If the stretch feels too intense, turn the toes under and raise the heels before grasping hold of them.
4. Keep pushing the thighs, hips, and abdomen forward, breathing deeply.
5. If you are strong enough, drop the head gently back so you are looking behind you. If you feel uncomfortable in the neck in any way, then ensure that you keep the head up and the eyes continue to look forward.
6. Keep breathing throughout.
7. Hold the pose for two to three full breaths.
8. To come out of the pose, lift the head if you have allowed it to drop backwards. Then release the left hand and move the weight of the body slowly over to the right before lifting up. Rise back up so that you are sitting on the knees, the toes are lying flat on the floor.
9. Breathe and relax

Precautions

Be cautious if you have any neck or back issues.

Contraindications

Do not practice this posture if you have a hernia. Do not drop the head back if you have neck issues. If you have severe back problems, do not attempt this posture. Seek expert advice.

Benefits

This pose can help to stimulate the nervous system because it provides compression to the spine. It improves flexibility in the neck and spine, and it can also assist with kyphosis and cervical spondylosis.

Connection Number

To be used in foreplay position #7.

Forward
Bend Pose

Legs Spread Back Stretch Pose (Pada Prasar Paschimottanasana)

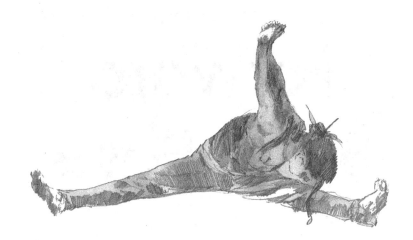

Legs Spread Back Stretch Pose (Pada Prasar Paschimottanasana)

1. Sit on your mat with the legs as wide apart as possible.
2. The hips are slightly tilting forward; the back is upright and straight.
3. Interlock the hands behind the back and straighten the arms, opening the chest.
4. This is a starting position as you will rotate to both the left and right.
5. Inhale, lifting the chest and turning towards the right leg. As you exhale, lower the head towards the knee and stretch the arms out behind you.
6. Hold for three to five breaths.
7. Inhale and lift to the central position and exhale.
8. Inhale, lifting the chest and turning towards the left leg. As you exhale, lower the head towards the left knee and stretch the arms out behind you.
9. Hold for three to five breaths.
10. Inhale up to the central position. Whilst exhaling, lower forward towards the mat. The aim is to try to reach the forehead to the floor directly in front of you, but do not force the body, or this will have an adverse effect. Raise the arms up behind you as high as possible.
11. Hold for three to five breaths.
12. Inhale as you come up to the starting position and exhale.
13. Release the arms and bring the legs in together.

Precautions

Be careful if you have hip, shoulder, or back issues other than those mentioned.

Contraindications

Those of you who may suffer with a slipped disc or sciatica should not practice this pose.

Benefits

This asana gives a stretch to the inside of the leg muscles as well as the hamstrings, and it increases flexibility in the hips. It extends the muscles between the shoulder blades. The entire abdominal and pelvic areas are massaged and toned, including the spleen, kidneys, pancreas, and adrenal glands. Excess weight to the central area is alleviated, as well as disorders affecting this region. The circulation system to the nerves and muscles of the spine are stimulated.

Connection Number

To be used in sexual positions #20 and #22 (reversed).

Relaxation
Poses

Extended Swan Pose (Utthita Hamsasana)

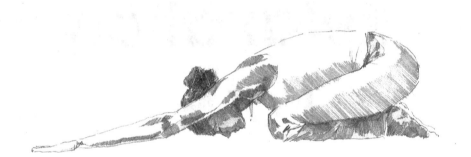

Extended Swan Pose (Utthita Hamsasana)

1. Kneel on the floor. Bring the buttocks to rest down onto the heels.
2. Relax the head down towards the knees or on the mat in front of you.
3. Whilst keeping the face looking down towards the floor, stretch the arms out in front of you with the palms of the hands lying flat on the ground.
4. Breathe and relax.

Precautions

Be cautious if you have any issues with the hips, back, or knees. For men, it may be a little more comfortable if you open the legs slightly.

Benefits

It relaxes the body, regulates the breath, and calms the mind.

Easy Pose (Sukhasana)

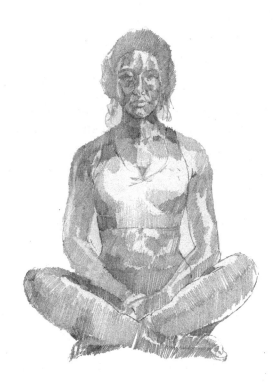

Easy Pose (Sukhasana)

1. Sit on the floor on the buttocks.
2. Cross the legs in a comfortable position.
3. Ensure that the back is straight; keep breathing slow and deeply.
4. Rest the hands comfortably on the knees.
5. Breathe and relax.

Precautions

Be cautious if you have any issues with the hips, back or knees.

Benefits

It relaxes the body, regulates the breath, and calms the mind.

Connection Number

To be used in foreplay position #5, #6 and sexual position #8.

Corpse Pose (Savasana)

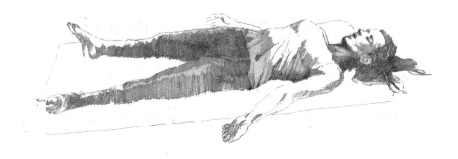

Corpse Pose (Savasana)

Description:

Lie flat on the ground facing upwards in the pose of a corpse (Sava). This posture is a relaxation pose. It removes tiredness, enabling the mind to settle and the whole body to relax. It can be carried out at the beginning of a practice if required, as well as the end. At the start of a session, it offers calmness to the mind and prepares you mentally and physically for the practice ahead.

Option One: For those with strong abdominal muscles.

1. Sit on your yoga mat with your arms stretched out in front of you.
2. Lower down vertebrae by vertebrae onto the mat, unfolding gradually until in a lying position. This ensures correct positioning of the hips and the base of the spine as you lie comfortably on the mat.
3. Relax the legs and separate the feet to hip width. Allow the feet to drop outwards to the sides and feel completely relaxed.
4. Rest the arms down by the side of you, with the hands approximately eight to ten inches away from the body. The palms should be facing upwards. Relax the shoulders down the back, opening gently across the chest.
5. Ensure that the chin is slightly tucked, bringing it towards the chest; this relieves pressure on the neck. Do not allow the chin to lift up, causing the head to tilt backwards.
6. Close the eyes and mouth, breathing only through the nose. Allow the breath to enter and leave the body naturally. Scan over the body to see if there is any tension held anywhere. If there is then breathe it away with each exhalation, release the pressure and let it go. Give up the weight of the body to the ground, relaxing deeper and deeper.

7. Watch and observe the breath, noticing each inhalation and exhalation. Take control of the breath as follows for a few minutes before letting go.

8. Inhale for three counts (this is one long inhalation counting 1 om, 2 om, 3 om)
Retain for one count (hold the breath for a count 1 om)
Exhale for four counts (this is one long exhalation counting 1 om, 2 om, 3 om, 4 om)

9. Relax. Stop controlling the breath and enjoy this comfortable, tranquil state.

Option Two: For beginners or those with weaker abdominal muscles.

1. Lie down flat on the back facing upwards.

2. Align the legs, back, and head, making sure you are not lying crooked.

3. Relax the legs and separate the feet to hip width. Allow the feet to drop outwards to the sides and feel completely relaxed.

4. Rest the arms down by your sides with the hands approximately eight to ten inches away from the body. The palms should be facing upwards. Relax the shoulders down the back, opening gently across the chest.

5. Ensure that the chin is slightly tucked, bringing it towards the chest; this relieves pressure on the neck. Do not allow the chin to lift up, causing the head to tilt backwards.

6. Close the eyes and mouth, breathing only through the nose. Allow the breath to enter and leave the body naturally. Scan over the body to see if there is any tension held anywhere. With each exhalation, release the pressure and let it go. Give up the weight of the body to the ground, relaxing deeper and deeper.

7. Watch and observe the breath, noticing each inhalation and exhalation. Take control of the breath as follows for a few minutes before letting go.
Inhale for three counts   1 om, 2 om, 3 om
Hold for one
Exhale for four counts   1 om, 2 om, 3 om, 4 om

8. Relax. Stop controlling the breath and enjoy this comfortable, tranquil state.

By keeping the hands slightly away from the body, your energy (prana) continues to flow around the body without restriction. If the hands are too far away, the energy link is broken down.

The relaxation outlined is based on observing the breath. There are various other relaxation techniques that can be used, such as tensing and relaxing each body part as you mentally focus on a specific area. Move around the entire body starting at either the head or feet, depending on your preference.

You may find that when the eyes are closed, you see varying colours. These can sometimes be related to the Chakra colours. During the relaxation period, watch as the colours change and different shapes are formed. The body will continue to relax whilst you observe.

In a class situation, some teachers mentally send you to a safe place that you conjure up from your imagination such as a beach, a garden, a mountain range or retreat of some other kind. Once established in your mind it can be accessed during times of stress to allow you to relax.

You will find that you enjoy some techniques more than others, but all options are positive because they prevent the mind from wandering off and thinking about all the jobs you have to do around the house, or your shopping list. Yoga is about the here and now and being in the moment.

Modification

Reversed corpse pose; lying on the front of the body with the forehead on the floor and the arms stretched out in front of you, is suitable for practitioners who suffer with slipped disc, stiff neck, and a stooping figure. You can use pillows if required to ensure that you are comfortable in the position. Alternatively, if able, use props under the knees and lie in a standard corpse pose. Pregnant women should lie on the left side using props, blankets, and blocks as necessary.

Connection Number

To be used in foreplay position #1 and sexual positions #17 and #22.

2

Setting the Mood

Make the Connection

There is nothing more special than the moment when the energies of two people connect. The electricity and adrenaline that pulses through your body creates excitement and a giddiness which cannot be compared to anything else. Each molecule racing through you ignites a deep passion inside as you gaze at each other through the gateway of your soul, the eyes. As you look lovingly at one another, the chemicals within you begin to flow.

Animal attraction is a primal instinct that connects human beings together, whatever your sexual preference. We are connected by emotions, desires, urges, passion, needs, and love, as well as the opposing negative attributes, but for the purpose of this book let us focus on the positive elements and how we can enjoy each other more.

In Tantric sex, it is said that the energy of the orgasm is prolonged by training the body through meditation, breathing techniques, and posture work. It is referred to in the Kama Sutra as Karezza, which is the term used to define a male's practice of pleasuring his partner and prolonging the intercourse by perpetuating his state of climax without actually ejaculating. Apparently it works through 'dry orgasms' (orgasms without ejaculation), which are pleasurable and still allows the sexual act to continue. Using these techniques heightens the enjoyment and satisfaction of the sexual experience for both parties.

If this is something that interests you then there are workshops and literature available to explain the techniques in more detail. Love Yoga has been designed on a more simplistic level in an easy to use format. It is a good starting point for individuals or couples who want to begin practising yoga or for those already participating. However, this book has the one added juicy ingredient; it connects lovers on a physical, mental and spiritual level whilst providing the benefits of getting fit and having fun in a pure and uncomplicated way.

Some people say that the connection between two people can be felt even if you are not in the same vicinity. You can feel when your partner is happy, upset, hurting, or angry. This does not always occur, so do not worry if this is not present in your relationship; it does not mean that the love you have for one another is any less. Everyone has an experience that is unique.

Whatever we believe, one fundamental fact remains; when the feelings are deep and passionate, consuming of our every thought, and if we feel that the second person makes us complete, then we refer to this person as a soul mate. A relationship is based on trust, full acceptance of each other, sharing emotions, supporting each others dreams, compromising when necessary and loving one another entirely. We are still able to fully function as an individual, but when togetherness occurs, both parties experience an unbreakable connection.

This experience is boundless to any sexual connotation or preference – love is love. Souls do not recognise gender, race, creed, or disability, only love. The benefit to this union is a lifetime of happiness. The shared kisses are magical and take us to places we have never been to before. If you are lucky enough to find true love then nothing else really matters.

Always remember to have fun with your partner and laugh, even during sex, but choose your moments. Obviously if you burst out laughing when he or she have just removed clothes, then that may be a little awkward. However, during foreplay and sometimes during sex, funny things occur, so share that moment and laugh. After all, it is love making, not an Oscar performance. Don't be too serious, or else it adds to the pressure. Sometimes it can help a person to relax and let go of inhibitions.

Have a lifetime filled with explicit joy!

Chakras

When your chakras are open, they link with the open chakras of another person; this draws you together on varying levels depending on which mirroring energy vortexes between you are open and emanating connectivity. This energy has no boundaries – it can be two men, two women, or a man and a woman.

The chakras are located within the astral body along the Shushumna, the central line of the body running from the perineum to the crown of the head. They are shown on the diagram below. The seven main spinning vortexes of subtle energy have individual properties that link with our physical body, senses and spirit having an effect on our whole being. They have a colour association, name, sound and rotate to their own vibrational rhythm. When blocked, the natural flow of energy is restricted around the body, and one can become imbalanced. Therefore it is suggested that the chakras are cleared on a regular basis. This can be achieved through yoga practice.

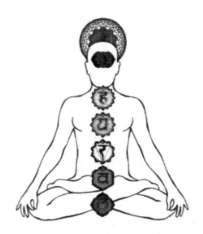

Outlined in the following table are basic facts about the seven chakras.

Chakra	Sanskrit	Location	Colour	Sense	Body	Effects
Root 1st	Muladhara Chakra (Root or support) Moo-lad-har-a	Base of the spine	Red	Smell	Lymph system, skeletal, elimination, central nervous system, nose, lower extremities	The root or base chakra is situated at the bottom of the spine at the perineum. The chakra is the closest out of the seven main chakras to the earth, making it the energetic gateway between us and earth, as well as the past, including our childhood. It is a grounding chakra and the seat of the Kundalini, or life force. When in balance, this chakra is associated with the physical aspects of our lives, our health and fitness, the survival instinct, and self-preservation. This is a masculine chakra connected with the solid elements of our body.

Chakra	Sanskrit	Location	Colour	Sense	Body	Effects
Sacral 2nd	Svadhisthana (Sweetness) Svaa-dhish-taa-na	Just below the navel	Orange	Taste	Sexual organs, reproductive system	The sacral or second chakra is located just below the navel and is in line with the fertility/sexual organs. It is the base of emotions associated with desire, sexual attraction, animal magnetism, vitality, creativity, and attraction. The second chakra is feminine. As it is one of the chakras associated with our emotions, there is the opportunity in balancing this chakra to deal with cleansing personality disorders involving instability, feelings of isolation, and an unbalanced sex drive. Therefore this chakra is very important in the connection between two people and feeling desirable.

Chakra	Sanskrit	Location	Colour	Sense	Body	Effects
Solar Plexus 3rd	Manipura (Lustrous gem) Mani-pura	Located between the sternum and the navel	Yellow	Sight	Solar plexus, muscles, skin, digestion, liver, eyes, face	The solar plexus or third chakra is associated with personal strength and is the power chakra. It is the fire of ambition and intellect, and it is also a base for various emotional outbursts such as joy, anger, over-sensitivity, low self-esteem, laughter, and the need to be in control. It is imperative to keep this chakra balanced because the emotion felt from here, if imbalanced, can be overwhelming. This chakra is known to be masculine.

Chakra	Sanskrit	Location	Colour	Sense	Body	Effects
Heart 4th	Anahata (Unstuck) Anaa-harta	Located at the centre of the chest	Green	Touch	Circulatory system, lungs, chest area	The fourth chakra at the heart is the linking chakra between the lower and higher chakras. The lower is the connection to earth, and the higher is the connection to the spiritual realm. It is filled with love, our understanding or foundation for relationships, the feeling of oneness, and our ability to lovingly connect to other people with compassion and without being judgmental. This is very much a feminine chakra.

Chakra	Sanskrit	Location	Colour	Sense	Body	Effects
Throat 5th	Vishuddha (Purification) Vish-u-ddha	Base of the neck	Blue	Hearing	Throat, neck, arms, hands, thyroid gland	The throat chakra is found at the base of the neck. This chakra is associated with our freedom of expression and our communicative aspect. It is our sound, our voice, and our inspiration in writing. It allows us to be heard. Our listening skills are also an element of this chakra because in order to be heard, you must also listen. This provides harmony and connection with others in our everyday lives. Through this chakra we activate our imagination and have the ability to dream. The fifth chakra is masculine.

Chakra	Sanskrit	Location	Colour	Sense	Body	Effects
Third eye 6th	Ajna (To perceive) Aaj-jnaa	Centre of the forehead	Indigo	Sensory Perception (ESP), clairvoyance, clairaudience	Forehead, temples, facial nerves, pituitary gland, endocrine system	The sixth chakra is situated at the third eye, which is in the centre of the brow and is known for connecting us with the spiritual realm and vision. Here we connect to our intuitional knowledge; through this chakra we are also able to look inside ourselves through turning the eye inwardly and surveying the inner self. We may experience extrasensory perception (ESP), inner sound, and clairvoyance. The sixth chakra is feminine.

Chakra	Sanskrit	Location	Colour	Sense	Body	Effects
Crown 7th	Sahasrara (Thousand fold, 1000 petal lotus) Sa-has-raa-ra	The very top of the head (crown)	Violet or White	Empathy	Brain, nervous system, pineal gland	The seventh and highest of the seven main chakras is situated at the crown of the head. The association here is with enlightenment, divine energy, higher intelligence, and self-realisation. The opening can take in cosmic energy and connect with the cosmic consciousness. It is said that at the time of death, prana (our life force energy) escapes through the seventh chakra, dispelling the connection between the physical and spiritual self. This chakra is masculine.

Love to Meditate

Set the atmosphere in the room. Light some candles that will be safe whilst you both have your eyes closed. Select meditative music that you both enjoy, and play it to create a calming ambience within the room. If you use crystals and have a number of rose quartz, known for its loving properties and connection to the heart chakra, create a circle using the crystals large enough for you both to sit in the centre. You will be facing one another in a comfortable, cross-legged pose; if this is not suitable, then rest in a kneeling position. You may be here for a while, so ensure that you will be comfortable.

For the purpose of the love meditation, you can be fully clothed in loose attire, in your favourite lingerie or underwear, or naked. Simply ensure that you are both content with the decision.

1. Sit close facing one another. Ensure that your back is straight and that you are breathing deeply throughout in and out of the nose.
2. Gently hold hands.
3. Look deeply into one another's eyes and really see the person in front of you: their purity, their good qualities and faults, their love and admiration for you, their honesty, and their commitment to you. They are your chosen life partner with whom you share your love and inner most secrets and desires. They are your friend, confidant, and lover.
4. Take it in turns to say one nice thing to each other. This will be part of your mantra, so remember their words. For example: 'You have beautiful eyes. Your smile warms my heart. You make me complete.'
5. Think of something nice about yourself. In order to love someone else, you must love yourself, or so they say. This may not be easy, but think positive thoughts about yourself and choose one to act as the second part of your mantra. Part one is your partner's comment. Part two is your kind thought towards yourself. These

will be repeated continuously and quietly in your head for the duration of the meditation.

6. Keep breathing.
7. Relax, listen to the calming music, look at the love in your partners eyes, breathe, and feel the electricity that you share as your hands touch. Both of you close your eyes and begin to repeat the mantras in your heads, repeating both parts slowly over and over again, meaning every word.
8. Allow yourselves to transcend. Imagine yourself out of your physical bodies. Imagine that you are pure energy and entwine the love you both have for each other to become one.
9. Relax in the loving company and breathe gently together.
10. Stay here, repeating the mantra for as long as you feel comfortable, but try for a minimum of five minutes. Slowly build up the length of time you can sit together in this way over a period of weeks.
11. This is intimacy without having to make a sexual connection. Take time to be together, share your love, and enjoy.

Sensory Pleasure

As a woman's energy emanates, the man receives messages sent from her spiritual being. As the energy connects, their desire for one another becomes heightened. They become lost in the moment, transcending to higher levels of desire whilst igniting a deep yearning for one another.

Visual

Begin by sitting opposite each other and gazing into one another's eyes. The closeness will begin to stir in the lower chakras. You don't always have time for long lengthy love sessions, but when you do, ensure you use the time wisely for one another to really connect.

You can be clothed in your favourite attire or lingerie, making it more tantalising when you strip. If you are both confident, then sit naked. The importance of this moment is for both of you to feel comfortable with yourself and your partner. You need to feel relaxed and contented whilst sitting opposite each other in this intense moment.

Continue to gaze deeply into their eyes, the soul's gateway, which is pure and coming only from a place of love. Take time to really look at each other and connect.

If you decide to take off your partner's clothing, take your time and enjoy slowly removing the garments whilst showing appreciation for their body as you look hungrily at their exposed skin.

If you decide to tease your partner by removing an item of clothing or by touching a part of your own body to create more excitement, then you must guide them with your eyes to the area. For example, if you decide to unbutton your blouse, look down towards the buttons as you slowly undo them; keep glancing back up at your partner's eyes to ensure they are enjoying what they see. Again take your time as this enhances and builds the excitement. The same rule applies if you are removing underwear.

Remember that this element is the preparation part, the time to build the excitement, so don't peak too soon.

Helpful Hints

Other suggestions can be as simple as watching a sexual movie together or looking through magazines and images. Do not be afraid to suggest your likes and dislikes, but be sensitive to your partner.

Perform a sexual act for your partner whilst they watch. This takes a huge amount of confidence and courage, so be patient. To excite them further, you could use sex toys, but whatever you decide to carry out for their viewing pleasure, you may want to have practised this in front of a mirror first so you know exactly what they are seeing and if you come across as sexy as you imagine, rather than wondering and being curious.

Send each other sexy images of yourselves throughout the day via text (or other messaging formats), setting the mood for the evening.

Dress up in your favourite lingerie (male or female) or sexy outfit and surprise them when they get home – or go to their place of work if you are brave enough.

Use mirrors so you can both see everything that is occurring. This can heighten the excitement as you both watch one another and enjoy looking at each other's bodies.

Talk (and Listen)

Talk to one another. Start over dinner, if this is your chosen activity for the evening, but then as the night progresses, allow the conversation to take a more intimate route. The subject of sex will probably come up as a topic of conversation anyway, because it's a favourite theme for most people.

During your closeness, open up and let your partner know your desires. Tell them what you want them to do to you, your fantasies, and your needs. As you begin to talk naughty and become aroused, the voice pitch changes, making it more seductive. The yearning for your partner comes across in your breathy tones. Explain how you like things to be carried out and guide their hands if necessary to help them understand what you really crave.

When you talk to each other, control your voice. Speak clearly, whisper some elements gently into their ear, and be seductive and sexy but not over the top. You still need to be true to yourself and one another.

Explain whilst emphasising words that heighten your pleasure. For example, "I really enjoy it when you *tease* my *clitoris slowly* with your *tongue* as you delicately *slide* your finger *in and out* of my wet *opening*."

Describe how they make you feel when they touch you in this way. Does your heart race? Does it make you gasp and take your breath away? Does it make you yearn for more? Does it make you want to scream and moan with desire? Does it make you thrash and writhe around? Or are you quietly excited, enjoying every sensation as you transcend to another level of pleasure?

Discover and learn how your body works and what it craves.

Most people know the famous book *Men Are from Mars and Women Are from Venus*. Some may agree that this is true, but during sex is where the connection happens. However, do not expect your partner to be telepathic. If you want something, ask for it. You may both learn something and realise that you are both a lot more open to trying new ideas than you ever contemplated.

Don't be afraid to express that you do not like something, even if it may be a fantasy of your partner's. A relationship is about compromise, so you could say that you may not be able to do all of it but are prepared to meet halfway. At least it shows consideration for their needs.

On the reverse of this, there may be times when your partner may not want to try, or even like, any of your suggestions. Do not be despondent or take offence. On a more positive note, you will make new discoveries between you which will enhance your sexual relationship, and you will discover more depth than you ever thought possible. Communication is the key.

When you do have time to talk to one another, ensure that you listen. Listening is an extremely important quality. We may not always find it easy, and our concentration can sometimes wander, but make the effort. After all, this is the love of your life.

Compliment personal details about your partner. Tell them how beautiful their eyes are and why. Are they emerald green and change to golden when the passion ignites inside them? Do they sparkle when they look at you? What about their back, legs, breasts, pectorals, stomach, hands, face, and all the physical elements? What is it about their body that you are really attracted to? Are they wearing something stunning? Explain why you like it. How does it compliment their shape? Is it the colour that suits them? What about their smile? Does it light up the room? How lustrous does their hair look? What are the wonderful qualities in their personality? Are they great parents and caring towards family and friends? Do you find them fascinating by the way they think and their level of intellect?

We are all complex, so take time to notice the subtle and the more obvious elements that constitute your chosen life partner.

During sex, do not be afraid to make a noise. It is perfectly natural to show your appreciation through vocal exclamations. Let yourself go. Your partner will soon be able to distinguish between your pleasure and ecstasy sounds, if they listen to the different tones and pitches of your moans. You will also learn each others sounds for when you are about to ejaculate or orgasm, which could be beneficial if you need to move out of the way before this occurrence happens.

Helpful Hints

Play a naughty game with one another that may involve reading out cheeky suggestions.

Read a naughty piece of literature to one another: an extract from a book, or something you found on the Internet or in a magazine. This could be something that you would like to act out with your partner, and it's a good way to introduce it into the relationship.

Create your own secret code that only each of you understand, outlining trigger words that have an alternative naughty meaning indicating to each other what is going to occur later when you are alone. It may lead to spontaneous sex whilst you are out and about.

Compliment each other throughout the day. Verbalise your thoughts – don't just keep it in your head. Say how attracted you are to them, being specific about their anatomy or personality and why you like that element of them.

Music is a universal language of connection that can be enjoyed by both parties. If the selection is made correctly, it can be soothing, and it may bring back memories of a moment in time that you may have shared at a concert or on a trip, which could spark happy discussions and create pleasurable memories of your life together. The right music may even set off your sexual trigger.

Touch

As you sit facing one another, gently begin to caress and feel the softness of the other person's skin, stroking every contour as you begin to trace each other with your hands and fingertips.

Start by touching the face, leaving an energetic sensation behind that the other person can continue to feel as you slowly move onto other areas of their body. Take your time slowly caressing every inch. Allow these pleasurable feelings to build as you connect deeper and deeper to one another.

As the nerve endings begin to awaken and respond, the desire for one another increases. After stroking your partner's face, slide your hand very slowly down the back of their neck, moving gently along one of their arms down to the fingers. Slowly massage each of the fingers from the base to the tip in a circular motion. Look into your partner's eyes for the duration of this.

Move onto the torso, which is a beautiful area for either a man or woman. The abdomen can be a particularly sensitive area for men. Do not touch any of the sensual areas; work around all of them, including the breasts and pectorals. This allows the discovery of other erogenous zones whilst the sexual regions become more sensitive and responsive and ache to be touched.

Whilst still avoiding the main sexual zones, stroke around the breasts and pectorals and follow the central line carefully moving down towards the belly button. Pause here and give it a tease with your finger. Continue down brushing over the front of the hips to the legs. Explore these with your fingers using massage and stroking techniques until you reach the back of the knees. Pay particular attention here before moving onto the lower leg prior to reaching the toes.

The nipples can be teased by circling them with your fingers around the areola (area around the nipple); they are sensitive for both men and women.

They can be stroked and tweaked between the first finger and thumb. The response is almost immediate: as the nipple reacts, it hardens, sending messages of pleasure to the brain.

As the vagina becomes receptive, it moistens around the opening, and the inner lip swells. The area changes as it responds to the fluctuation in hormone levels flowing through the body. These visible and apparent transformations inform her partner that she wants him and is ready to receive his erect penis deep inside her.

The male reaction to desire is more obvious. His penis becomes erect and enlarges in size, ready to be welcomed into the warm, moist vaginal opening.

Both of these areas need to be fully explored with gentle strokes and massaging actions of the fingers. The clitoris can be massaged in a circular motion. Ensure that the clitoris is moist as you continue teasing; this heightens the pleasure and increases the sensation. You will see as your partner's body becomes stimulated. She will naturally respond to your delicate touch. If she is lying down, the back may arch, the hips will gently thrust, and the muscles around the vagina pulsate as excitements runs through each cell.

Women also ejaculate. This can be a little more extreme and messy than when a man ejaculates, but she should release and let go. Love is meant to be fair and equal. It is important for both parties to find satisfaction.

To tease the penis, start by stroking its full length up and down. Each time you reach the tip, circle your finger around the area. Whilst doing this, take the scrotum in your other hand if possible and massage it playfully but carefully.

Slide the foreskin back and forth to stimulate your partner further, but be careful not to get him too excited. Start off slow and then quicken the pace if he requests. Find out what kind of pressure he prefers by tightening and loosening your grip.

As your partner relaxes and enjoys the sensation, take the hand that is massaging the gonads and slide your finger to caress the perineum. If your partner is feeling a little more adventurous, slide your finger up to the anus but only if he is absolutely comfortable, then insert the finger gently but quite deep into the anus. Provided that both parties are agreeable, move it back and forth. There is an area in here which is like a trigger that can cause the man to cum, which gives him a completely different sensation to ejaculating generally. Please ensure that you both feel happy, safe, and relaxed. You should take your time.

Ensure that you are always careful and tender, unless your partner requests or you both agree otherwise.

Helpful Hints

Use props to enhance the sensation of touch, such as a silk scarf or feather to gently caress the body.

You could use the head of a flower to stroke along exposed skin.

Try using ice because it creates an instant reaction. Circle it slowly around the nipple. Watch their body respond with pleasure.

Use oil to massage each other, creating a slippery surface between the two of you, heightening the sensation and making manoeuvrability easier as you fully connect on a sexual level.

If you are comfortable, you could bring a vibrator into the bedroom (or whichever room you choose) as a pleasure tool for both of you. Investigate other love accessories.

If you like wine (or another tipple), take a sip into your mouth and then slowly kiss your partner, transferring some of the wine to them so that you can both enjoy it.

Smell

Ensure that personal hygiene is taken care of and your body is well groomed. Clothing must be clean and presentable to entice your partner. Wear aftershave or perfume if you desire, although natural, clean bodily aroma is nature's way of attracting your mate. Again, this is where the animal instincts come into action. Each of us has a unique odour as desire oozes out of our pores. The opposing person connects to this animal magnetism and it draws them in, making it the perfect formula for fun.

Burn incense to set the mood in the room. Obviously do not use too much because it can be extremely strong, and don't use a scent that may remind you of elsewhere (for example, the same incense that your yoga teacher uses at the studio). You need to only associate the chosen incense with your sensual fun and playful activities. This creates relaxation and opens the senses. Ensure also that you both like it.

Use scented massage oils, taking your time to carefully massage your partner from head to toe in turn. Allow the aromatherapy scents to relax and soothe away any cares so that your time together is calm and pleasurable.

Helpful Hints

Make sure that the chosen area in which you are about to enjoy your sexual encounter is a clean, uncluttered, and gently lit environment where you will not be disturbed.

Make sure if you are using a bed for fun and are going to sleep in it afterwards, it is clean and fresh.

Have a soothing but fun bubble bath together. Enjoy washing and caressing each other, allowing your hands to gently wander exploring every region of their naked body. If you don't like hot baths, take a shower together and enjoy the same pleasurable sensations.

Taste

We all have a unique blend of elements that make us taste differently to anyone else. The individuality of this manifested combination is the reason that we are attracted to some people and not others. This is our bodily scent, which is primal. We can try to mask it with perfume and soaps, but it will still remain. It is known as animal attraction on a subconscious level.

For this section, I am suggesting using the lips and tongue instead of the fingers to tease your partner. Trying this may not suit everyone, but it is very pleasurable.

Instead of using the fingertips, trace the tongue along and around the areas of the body, incorporating gentle nibbling and sucking. The performing of this ritual is both satisfying for the recipient as well as the giver. This is precious time together, so do not rush; embrace each moment.

If you are pleasing a woman, when you reach the vaginal area, tease the clitoris whilst simultaneously inserting a finger into the vaginal opening, moving it back and forth whilst the tongue plays in a circular motion with the clitoris. The woman will find it very difficult to keep control. Enjoy the taste and take satisfaction from hearing her cry out with excitement.

Take time to pleasure your man. Tease the penis by licking up and down the shaft as well as around the base and the top. Continue circling the tip of the penis with your tongue as you draw the foreskin gently back and forth with one hand, massaging the gonads with the other. After a while hold onto the base of the penis with one hand and take the full length of the erect penis in your mouth, moving up and down whilst gently sucking. Start off slowly and quicken the pace if your partner prefers this. Keep the pressure constant and not too strong, but ensure that the teeth are kept away, preventing them from catching the organ.

It may be worth considering whether you have an issue if your partner ejaculates when you are performing a sex act, not all people enjoy this experience. If you feel this way, then during your time together talking, explain how you feel and request that they give you a subtle signal prior to ejaculation so that you can considerately move away. Bodily fluids can be ingested, but this is down to personal preference, and not everyone enjoys this process.

Helpful Hints

Sit facing each other in the kitchen, both of you undressed or in an item that you don't mind spoiling. Have an array of food in front of you. One of you is to be blindfolded whilst you are fed from the different foods and then you swap. Amongst the feeding, leave room for plenty of kisses and sensual caressing. Remember that the feelings of the person blindfolded are heightened because they do not know what to expect as they cannot see what is about to occur.

3

Creating the
Union of Love

The Entwined Collection – Two People with a Desire for Yoga and Each Other

Some of the classical postures may have been adapted slightly to enable the foreplay and love making to occur more comfortably. Some of the postures are quite difficult, but continued practice will build strength in the physical body. Not all postures from section one are used in the latter part of this book, but feel free to try your own sexual blends using the asanas.

Love is a journey. Along the way it is important to create lots of happy memories and many loving and caring times. Have fun and enjoy every minute you spend together. Life is not always a bed of roses, and at times we all become fraught and fractious, sometimes for no apparent reason. Life is short and love is precious, and our time for each other can become minimal, especially with working hard and our social commitments. It gets even tougher if you are blessed with children at some point. We are all guilty of forgetting that, so grasp every moment when you can. Remember to laugh, and always try to recall why you fell in love in the first place.

No one said that love is easy, and it is something that needs to be worked on and handled with care. However, the following ideas may offer a little bit of spice to keep the connection between two lovers strong.

Foreplay

#1 Crow and Corpse Pose

This is suitable for either person to be lying underneath (corpse) or in the upper position (crow) so that both of you can experience the pleasure. Crow is a difficult pose, so be cautious, and obviously be sure that you are capable of accomplishing the asana before carrying it out above your partner. The idea here is to tease your partner's genitalia as they sit above you in anticipation.

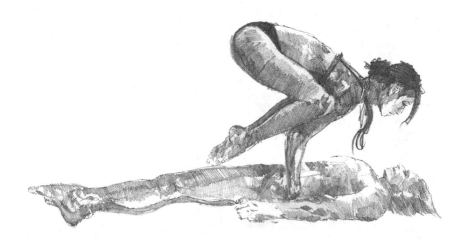

#2 Boat and Cobra Pose

As you sit in boat pose, you are exposing yourself and opening up your genitalia to be teased by your partner as they rest in front of you in a low cobra pose (or sphinx pose, if that is more comfortable and stable). Enjoy being teased. This can be enjoyed by either party. It is wise to rest the arms behind you if in boat pose for stability.

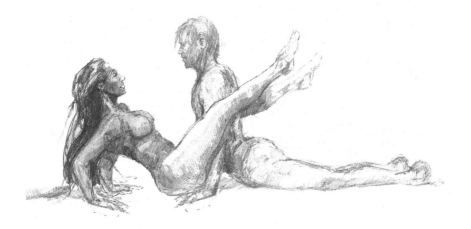

#3 Tree and Mountain Pose

Stand in the beautiful tree pose, opening the arms into blossoming tree pose if you wish. Allow yourself to be free and open to your loved one as they caress your body, investigating every part of you with their hands as they stand in the strong mountain pose.

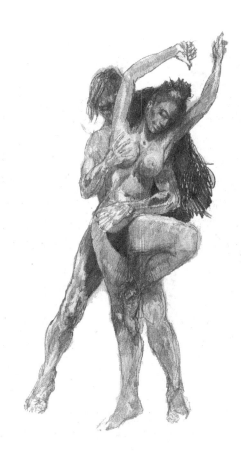

#4 Mountain and Shoulder Stand Pose

As you achieve the shoulder stand pose, try to relax one of your legs away, exposing yourself to your partner and enabling them to have the freedom to pleasure you as they stand in a sturdy mountain pose. Do not stay in these postures for too long, but do try them if you feel able, and enjoy the occasion.

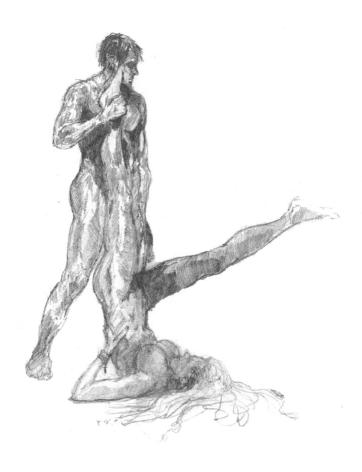

#5 Crescent Moon and Easy Pose

As you perform this wonderful posture (crescent moon), stretch and sink deeply into the asana. Your partner is free to excite you whilst they sit comfortably in front of you (easy pose), giving you pleasure.

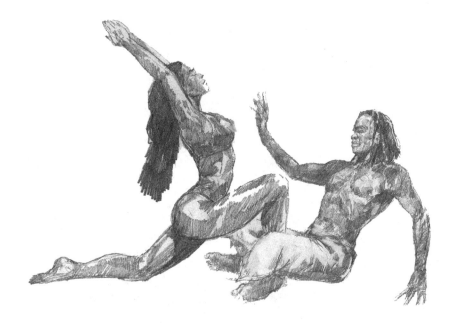

#6 Extended Hand to Big Toe and Easy Pose

Stand in this strong pose (extended hand to big toe pose) with caution, particularly when you begin to feel stimulation as your partner gives you pleasures whilst sitting in front of you (easy pose). Enjoy the intimacy but remember that this is just an appetiser.

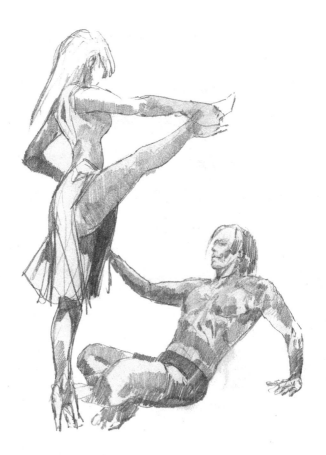

#7 Camel and Cobra Pose

To enhance your foreplay, either you or your partner can come into the camel pose whilst your partner satisfies you and performs the cobra pose, giving them the ability to be close to you. The sensation is heightened due to the genitalia being pushed forward in the pose. Remember that this is the foreplay section – there is plenty more to come, so take your time.

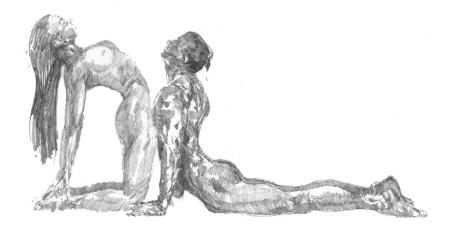

Sexual Connection

#8 Pigeon and Easy Pose

This beautiful connection can be made through combining the two poses together. It can be a little tricky, but once you accomplish the combination, the union you will feel is both satisfying and exquisite.

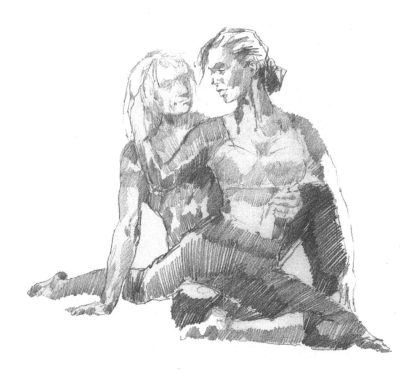

#9 Dancer and Mountain Pose

These poses combined together are beautiful. It allows the male party to be very close and both parties can reach a high level of pleasure.

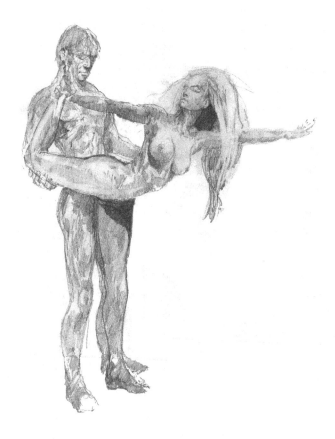

#10 Shoulder Stand and Warrior I Pose

Start in a mountain pose to create the initial position, as per the first image, before moving into the more difficult combination of the shoulder stand and warrior pose. Be careful when moving into the more complicated position as you will notice, the male is astride the female which can be a little awkward to achieve. The penetration here is very intense. Feel the connection between you both. Take your time and be gentle as you move back and forth in a slow, rhythmic way. Do not stay here for too long as both poses are strong.

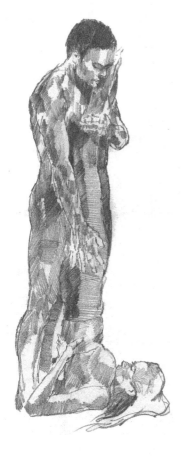

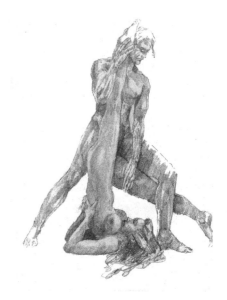

#11 The Cobbler Combination

Connecting in comfortable positions can be very pleasurable as well as surprisingly liberating, because as you start in the easier options, it will give you a taste to move onto the more involved pose combinations. Feel free to express yourself to your partner and relish the intimacy that you share in these moments together. This is a wonderful, close fusion that everyone can enjoy.

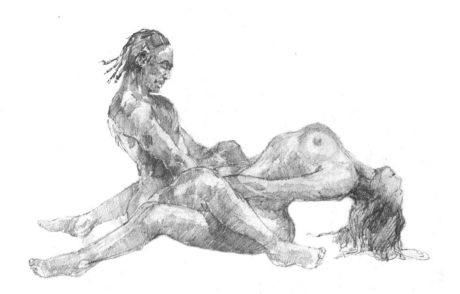

#12 Bridge Pose

As with the foreplay, the sensation here for the woman in the bridge pose is heightened due to the clitoris pushing up and forward as the penetration occurs. This can cause a woman to orgasm quickly, so take your time. Start slowly and listen to the sounds of pleasure coming from your partner as an indicator to her level of pleasure so you can take your time and not let her peak too soon.

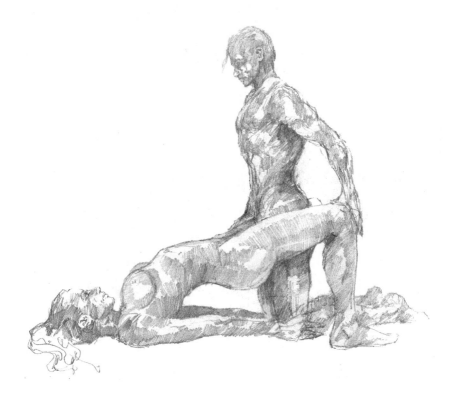

#13 Triangle Pose (Both Parties)

These poses entwine together to give a sensual feeling to both participants. Enjoy the beauty and fluidity of these poses as you connect to one another on a deep, spiritual, and loving level.

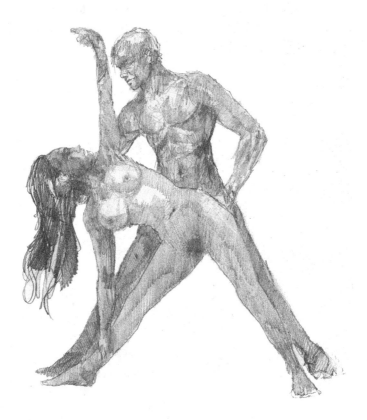

#14 Wheel and Mountain Pose

As your partner moves into the difficult pose of the wheel, move in between her legs and penetrate her gently as you stand in the strong, supportive asana of mountain. Give her support as you carefully hold her. Take care because the wheel pose is very strong, so this may not be a connection that you can endure extensively, but you can take pleasure from it nonetheless. Do not be put off due to the complexity of the image.

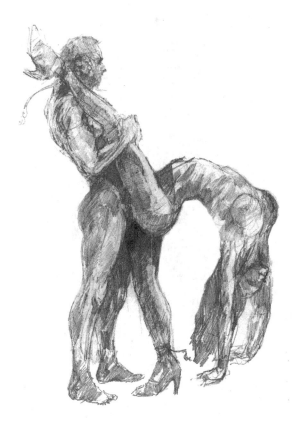

#15 Warrior Creation

This strong link between two people is intense and thrilling. The physical strength of both parties during the closeness as well as the mental connection is powerful and energetic. Lust oozes out of every pore and chemicals flow like electricity around the body as this deep relationship manifests.

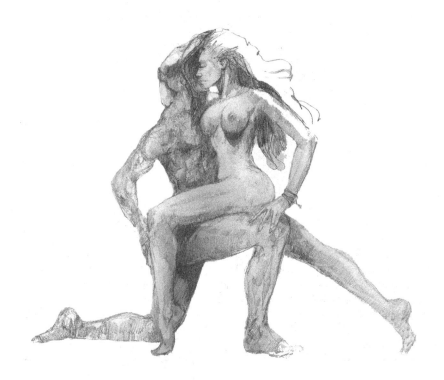

#16 Downward Facing Dog (Extended Leg) and Warrior I Pose

These poses, combined together, give deep pleasure for both parties. When you are in downward facing dog, extend one of your legs behind you, allowing your partner to gently take hold of it and offer you support. Work carefully with your partner as they penetrate you from behind. Push back as your partner pushes forward, and between you create a rhythmic pace that is comfortable for you both. Remember that these asanas are very strong, so do not hold them for a prolonged period of time.

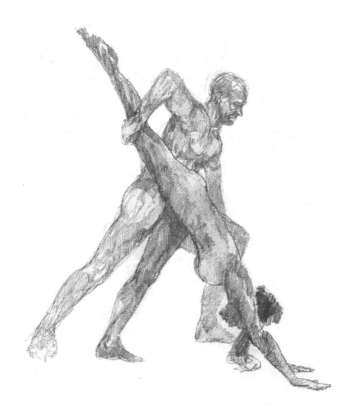

#17 Corpse and Plank Pose

This is essentially the missionary position, but it is a classical position that can still be enjoyed by both parties. The simplicity and closeness of the position is wonderful to keep you both connected.

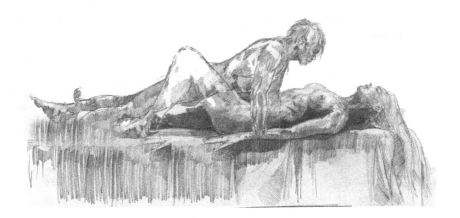

#18 Cobbler and Plank Pose

Lie back and relax with your legs in cobbler pose, allowing the knees to fall out to the side and opening yourself to your partner as he uses the strength in his arms to position himself over you in plank pose. This simple combination will give you both closeness and enjoyment.

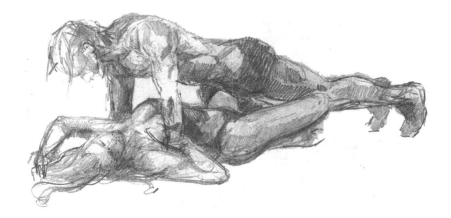

#19 Forward Bend and Mountain Pose

These poses are taken from the beautiful sequence of the sun salutation, but these can be used aside from the sequence to enable the exploration of a little sexual pleasure. This combination is simple and fun.

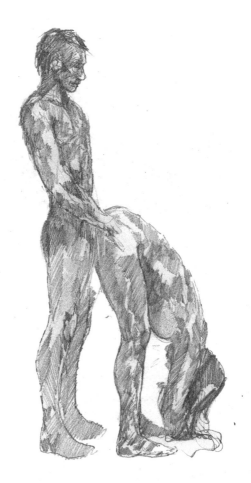

#20 Legs Spread Back Stretch Pose (Both Parties)

Enjoy the closeness and sensual feeling of this combination as you sit together. Move purposefully and slowly as you look into each other's eyes, allowing the love connection to flow. As you sit on top of your male partner, if you are flexible enough, you could raise one or both of your legs and bring them to rest on your partner. Take time to discover your own way of performing this.

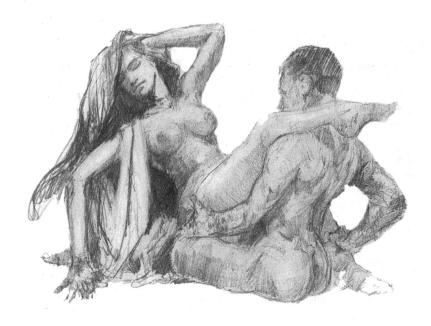

#21 Boat and Cobra Pose

Use your arms to support yourself in the boat pose. That will give these connecting poses some longevity because the boat pose can be quite difficult to hold. The beauty of these postures shows in the contour lines as the bodies interact, creating a union of ecstasy.

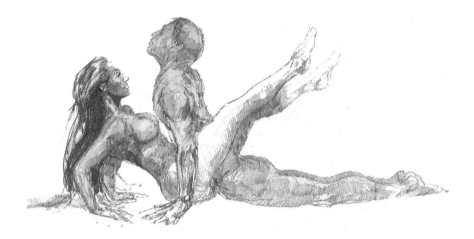

#22 Corpse and Legs Spread Back Stretch Pose (Reversed)

Even though you may be sat facing the opposite way to your partner (legs spread back stretch pose) as he lays back (corpse pose), you can turn slightly to look at him as you both enjoy every moment of the pleasure being received. To change the connection, slightly come up from corpse pose into a higher position resting on the elbows or seated, bringing you both even closer in your union.

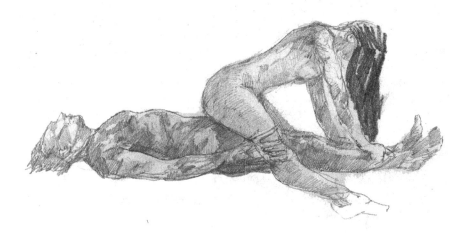

#23 Mountain and Extended Hand to Big Toe Pose

This combination can be quite difficult because it places a lot of pressure on the legs in both mountain and the pose where the leg is raised. However, if you can achieve this arrangement, then you will both feel a lot of pleasure.

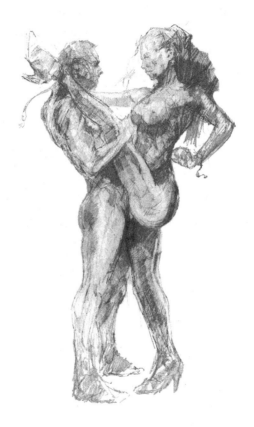

About the Author

I am a qualified yoga teacher and holistic therapist including certification in counselling. I have personally trained in various forms of yoga for over 15 years undertaking numerous workshops and continued development. The sexual element to this book is included because this is something else that I and many other people enjoy so I have created a union of both subjects together enabling others to experience pleasure on all levels from passion for yoga to desire for each other. I am lucky enough to have found love in my life, I have a wonderful husband and two amazing children who I live with in Derbyshire in the UK. My life is happy and fulfilled, my aim is to help others find completion by loving themselves through yoga and each other through sexual connection and this book has been created to give everyone who has an interest a helping hand.

Original hand drawn sketches by Jaye a UK based artist specialising in yoga posture drawings and who is also a qualified yoga teacher.

Printed in the United States
By Bookmasters